THE
BARBARA KRAUS
FAT COUNTER

OTHER BOOKS BY BARBARA KRAUS

The Barbara Kraus International Cookbook
The Dictionary of Sodium, Fats, and Cholesterol
The Barbara Kraus Calorie Counter
The Barbara Kraus Cholesterol Counter
The Barbara Kraus 30-Day Cholesterol Program
Calories & Carbohydrates
Complete Guide to Sodium
Barbara Kraus Calorie Guide
Barbara Kraus Carbohydrate Guide
Barbara Kraus Complete Guide to Sodium
Barbara Kraus Sodium Guide to Brand Names & Basic Foods

THE
BARBARA KRAUS
FAT COUNTER

Barbara Kraus

THE BODY PRESS/PERIGEE

The Body Press/Perigee Books
are published by
The Putnam Publishing Group
200 Madison Avenue
New York, NY 10016

Library of Congress Cataloging-in-Publication Data

Kraus, Barbara.
The Barbara Kraus fat counter / Barbara Kraus.
p. cm.
ISBN 0-399-51715-4 (trade paperback) :
1. Food—Fat content—Tables. I. Title. II. Title: Fat counter.
TX551.K678   1992   91-25457 CIP
641.1′4—dc20

Cover design by Bob Silverman

Printed in the United States of America
3   4   5   6   7   8   9   10

*To Ted Materna and
heart patients everywhere.*

INTRODUCTION

This volume lists the total fat and the saturated and unsaturated fatty acid content of several thousand food items. In recent years these nutrients have been receiving increasing attention by nutritionists and the medical profession because of their possible relationship to obesity and to coronary heart disease (atherosclerosis). Of course, diet is not the only factor to be considered in heart disease. Other considerations are high blood pressure; heredity, for instance, genetic regulation of blood cholesterol and lipids; cigarette smoking; lack of exercise; stress; and certain ailments such as diabetes.

There are various forms of fat—saturated, unsaturated, and polyunsaturated. As a rule of thumb, fats are saturated if they are solid at room temperature. If they are liquid at room temperature, they are invariably unsaturated. While this is a general rule and there are exceptions to it, it is useful as a practical guide. A great many foods contain both kinds of fat in varying proportions. Oils from fish and plants provide the most abundant amounts of polyunsaturated fats, the types that are largely free of hydrogenation. Coconut oil is an exception. It is high in saturated fats and solid at room temperature.

Meats, cheeses, eggs, and most animal products are high in saturated fatty acids. The listings in this book showing the values for unsaturated fatty acids include both monounsaturated and polyunsaturated fats. At present the information available for many foods is still not adequate to give a complete breakdown of these two forms of fat. New federal requirements for labeling commercial products should result in more complete information in the near future, and later editions of this book will keep abreast of such new information.

ARRANGEMENT OF THIS BOOK

Foods are listed alphabetically by brand name or by the name of the food. The singular form is used for the entries, that is, blackberry instead of blackberries. Most items are listed individually although a few are grouped (see p. 10). For example, all candies are listed together so that if you are looking for *Mars* bar, look first under Candy, then under *M* in alphabetical order. But if you are looking for a breakfast food such as oatmeal, you will find it under *O* in the main alphabet. Many cross references are included to assist you in finding items known by different names.

Under the main headings, it is often not possible nor even desirable to follow an alphabetical arrangement. For basic foods such as apricots, the first entries are for the fresh product weighed with seeds as it is purchased in the store, then the fruit in small portions as they may be eaten or measured. These entries are followed by the processed products, canned (although it may actually be a bottle or a jar), dehydrated, dried, and frozen items. This basic plan, with adaptations where necessary, was followed for fruits, vegetables, and meats.

In almost all entries, where data were available, the U.S. Department of Agriculture figures are shown first. The USDA values represent averages from several manufacturers and are shown for comparison with the values from individual companies, or for use where particular brands are not available.

All brand-name products have been italicized and company names appear in parentheses.

PORTIONS USED

The portion column is a most important one to read and note. Common household measures are used wherever possible. For some items, the amounts given are those commonly purchased in the store, such as one pound of meat or a 15-ounce package of cake mix. These quantities can be divided into the number of servings used in the home and the nutritive values in each portion can then be readily determined. Any ingredients added in preparing such products must also be taken into the final tally.

The smaller portions given are for foods as served or measured in moderate amounts, such as ½ cup of reconstituted juice, or 4 ounces of meat. Be sure to adjust the amount of the nutrients to the actual portions you use. For example, if you serve one cup of juice instead of ½ cup, multiply the amount of the nutrients shown for the smaller measure by two.

The size of portions you use is extremely important in controlling the intake of any nutrient. The amount of a nutrient is directly related to the weight of the food served. The weight of a volumetric measure, such as a cup or a pint, may vary considerably depending on many factors; 4 ounces by weight may be very different from ½ cup or 4 fluid ounces. Ounces in the tables are always ounces by weight unless specified as fluid ounces, fractions of a cup, or other volumetric measures. Foods that are fluffy in texture, such as flaked coconut and bean sprouts, vary greatly in weight per cup, depending on how tightly they are packed. Such foods as canned green beans also vary when measured with and without liquid; for instance, canned beans with liquid weigh 4.2 ounces for ½ cup, but drained beans weigh 2.5 ounces for the same ½ cup. Check the weights of your serving portions regularly. Bear in mind that you can reduce or increase the intake of any nutrient by changing the serving size.

It is impossible to convert all the portions to a uniform basis. Some sources were able to report data only in terms of weight, with no information on cup or other volumetric measures. We have shown small portions in quantities that might reasonably be expected to be served or measured in the home or institution.

You will find in the portion column the phrases "weighed with bone" and "weighed with skin and seeds." These descriptions apply to the products as you purchase them in the markets, but the nutritive values shown are for the amount of edible food after you discard the bone, skin, seed, or other inedible parts. The weight given in the measure or quantity column is to the nearest gram or fraction of an ounce.

Data on the composition of foods are constantly changing for many reasons. Better sampling and analytical methods, improvements in marketing procedures, and changes in formulas of mixed products may alter values for all of the nutrients. Weights of packaged foods are frequently changed. It is essential to read label information in order to be knowledgeable about these matters and to make intelligent use of food tables.

OTHER NUTRIENTS

These tables are not intended as a dietary guide. Any drastic change from a normal, varied diet should be undertaken only under the guidance of a qualified physician. Do not forget that other nutrients—protein, carbohydrates, minerals, and vitamins—are extremely important in diet planning. From a nutritional viewpoint, perhaps the best advice that can be given is to eat a varied diet with all classes of food represented. Meat, fish, chicken, fats and oils, milk, vegetables, fruits, and grain products are all important sources of essential nutrients, and some foods from each of these classes should be included every day.

If you have been medically advised to control your intake of one or more nutrients shown in these tables, with your doctor's guidance you can choose those foods that will fit your specific needs and also provide an acceptable yet varied selection. Control of certain nutrients, such as cholesterol or saturated fat, need not condemn you to a monotonous diet. There is a rich and varied assortment of foods in our markets that will meet any medical requirement. Choose wisely and eat well.

SOURCES OF DATA

Values in this dictionary are based on publications issued by the U.S. Department of Agriculture and on data submitted by manufacturers and processors. The U.S. Department of Agriculture issues basic tables on food composition for use in the United States. The commercial products from USDA publications represent average values obtained on products of more than one company. The figures designated as "home recipe" are based on recipes on file with the Department of Agriculture. Data on commercial products listed by brand name in this publication are based on values supplied by manufacturers and processors for their own individual products. Supermarket brand names, such as A&P's *Ann Page,* or private labels, could not be included in this book inasmuch as they are not usually analyzed under these trade names. Every care has been taken to interpret the data and the descriptions supplied by the companies as fully and as accurately as possible. Many values have been recalculated to different portions from those submitted, in order to bring about greater uniformity among similar items.

The values for saturated and unsaturated fats are rounded to the nearest whole number. Therefore, the individual constituents may add up to more or less than the figure given for total fat. In many cases, the values for unsaturated fat were derived by the subtraction of the amount of saturated fat from the total fat. In a very few instances, manufacturers reported saturated and unsaturated fat analyses that did not add up to the total fat shown. This minor discrepancy occurred because, in their opinion, the undetermined fatty acids were present in insignificant amounts.

Analysis of foods to provide information on nutritive values are extremely expensive to conduct. Many small companies cannot afford to have their products analyzed and were unable to provide data or were able to provide only a portion of the data requested. Other companies have simply never gotten around to having the analyses done. New requirements for labeling nutritive values for products may provide information on additional items in the future. Wherever data were unavailable, blank spaces are left, which may be filled in by the reader at a later time.

FOODS LISTED BY GROUPS

Foods in the following classes are reported together rather than as individual items in the main alphabet: bread, cake, cake icing, cake icing mix, candy, cheese, cookies, cookie mix, crackers, gravy, pie, pudding or pie filling, salad dressing, soft drinks, soup.

BARBARA KRAUS

FOREWORD

In describing an Eskimo banquet, Hans Ruesch wrote in *Top of the World* that they alternated the sweet bear meat with green, moldy marrow and rank tallow that they washed down with swills of tea, careful not to touch fish while eating meat, lest they should arouse the ire of the spirits.

The eating of meat and fish together as part of the same dish—or the prohibitions against doing so—constitute a fascinating glimpse into some cultural patterns that began in prehistory and extend to the present day. One Roman emperor, Vitellius, is said to have sent out a whole fleet to scour the Mediterranean coasts for the ingredients of a dish consisting of flamingo tongues, pike livers, pheasant brains, and lamprey milt.

Numerous Roman dishes combined meat and fish. That habit persisted in many parts of the world. It spread throughout Europe, including Scandinavia, and is apparent in the culinary preferences of Africans, South Americans, and Chinese, but not in the native cuisines of the Japanese or the Americans.

Thus, except for the anchovy in your Caesar salad, it is virtually impossible to think of an indigenous American recipe combining meat and fish. It was fascinating to observe the reactions of a sampling of Americans knowledgeable about foods when asked to cite recipes with a meat-fish combination. They pondered for a long moment, then named paella and antipasto, both foreign dishes.

Of course, there is no one simple explanation for the eating preferences of all peoples at all times. As society changes, so do our dining habits. In many parts of the world, dietary patterns are being reshaped as specific nutrients receive increasing attention by nutritionists and the medical profession because of their possible relationship to atherosclerosis (coronary heart disease). This concern includes an examination of the role of total fat in the diet, covering both saturated and unsaturated fatty acids, as well as cholesterol and sodium.

Patients with coronary disease and high blood pressure are often placed on diets in which one or more of these nutrients is controlled. Of course, diet is not the only factor to be considered in heart disease. Physicians now believe that the conditions leading to early heart attacks are the result of a lifetime of habits that predispose individuals to such attacks. Many now recommend that certain changes in dietary patterns be made in early childhood.

Barbara Kraus

UPDATE ON FAT IN YOUR DIET

As Barbara Kraus noted in the foreword to this volume, culturally in-grained dietary patterns are changing at an unprecedented rate in many parts of the world as nutrition research continues to unveil the close links between the foods we choose and impaired health, particularly heart disease.

In the last several years, nutritionists have been scrutinizing the intake of fats by Americans and other populations with a diet rich in red meats and dairy products. Their research now strongly suggests that unsound eating habits, often acquired early in life, may lay the basis for the onset of various nutrition-linked diseases in later years, sometimes even in people under forty. The latest recommendations, therefore, apply not only to adults but also to children age two or older.

As of 1991, the United States Department of Agriculture urges that no more than 30 percent of what we eat be in the form of fat, and that only 10 percent of those calories consist of saturated fatty acids. Thus, not only how much fat we consume but also the type can determine how healthy we remain.

Presently, up to as much as 50 percent of the calories consumed by a great many Westernized societies is in the form of fat, and much of that is often the saturated type, the kind your body may transform into choles-terol. And it is cholesterol that tends to deposit on arteries and impair blood flow, thus leading to heart attacks.

In simplest terms, fats fall into three types. Saturated fats, which if present in excessive amounts can lead to a rise in cholesterol, are present in some of the most popular traditional foods throughout the world. These are beef, pork, butter, whole milk, and cocoa butter (choco-late), as well as a few vegetable sources, such as coconut oil and palm oil. In general, organ meats, for instance, liver and brains, whether from beef or pork, are particularly high in saturated fat and should be used very sparingly even in the normal diet.

The other types of fat (monounsaturated and polyunsaturated) pose less of a health risk. The monounsaturated type is present in virtually all foods of animal origin and in a few vegetable products as well. Monoun-saturated fats can help reduce the levels of certain forms of cholesterol. For example, the chief monounsaturated oil from olives is oleic acid. It has been shown to reduce certain forms of cholesterol by as much as 15 percent. Oils from peanuts and avocados are also monounsaturated. Linoleic acid, the major constituent in polyunsaturated fats, the kind not transformed into cholesterol, is present in corn, soy, cottonseed, safflower, and sunflower oils. It, too, has been shown to lower one form of cholesterol by up to 15 percent.

The third type of fat, the polyunsaturated kind, is desirable since it is *not* transformed into cholesterol. This type comes largely from vegetables. Therefore, whenever possible, it's preferable to use safflower, sunflower, corn, soybean, and cottonseed oils rather than butter or the hydrogenated fat products, such as lard or the solid fats often used as shortening. Some fish oils are also polyunsaturated. This is why heart patients and those who are obese often are advised to eat more fish rather than red meats.

It has long been known that fat is a prime source of energy that is released more slowly than the "quick pickup" we get from carbohydrates. However, on a gram-for-gram basis, fats provide considerably more calories than do either carbohydrates or proteins. The following comparison of what is known as the *fuel factor* shows why a high-fat diet can quickly add on unwanted pounds:

1 gram protein	=	4 calories
1 gram carbohydrate	=	4 calories
1 gram fat	=	9 calories

But a word of caution: Fats are essential in normal human metabolism. A totally fat-free diet would also prove harmful. A normal diet supplies some essential fatty acids that our own organs cannot manufacture, and provides a natural storehouse of fat-soluble vitamins (A, D, E, and K).

As Dr. Alan Beckles of New York City's Beth Israel Medical Center points out in *The Barbara Kraus 30-Day Cholesterol Program,* "Our dietary habits are generally poor as they relate to fat consumption. . . . Americans need to be pushed to change their lifestyle when it comes to dietary habits. We need to make these changes for ourselves and especially for future generations."

To help you achieve that goal, this new volume on the fat content of many of the most common foods makes it easier to determine exactly how much fat, including the saturated type, may be in the food items on your shopping list or in the dishes you select in a restaurant.

Margaret Markham

ABBREVIATIONS AND SYMBOLS

* = prepared as package directs[1]
< = less than
& = and
" = inch
canned = bottles or jars as well as cans
dia. = diameter
fl. = fluid
liq. = liquid
lb. = pound
med. = medium

oz. = ounce
pkg. = package
pt. = pint
qt. = quart
sq. = square
T. = tablespoon
Tr. = trace
tsp. = teaspoon
wt. = weight

All foods not identified by company or trademark brand name have data based on material obtained from the United States Department of Agriculture or Health, Education and Welfare-Food and Agriculture Organization.

EQUIVALENTS

By Weight

1 pound = 16 ounces
1 ounce = 28.35 grams
3.52 ounces = 100 grams

By Volume

1 quart = 4 cups
1 cup = 8 fluid ounces
1 cup = ½ pint
1 cup = 16 tablespoons
2 tablespoons = 1 fluid ounce
1 tablespoon = 3 teaspoons
1 pound butter = 4 sticks or 2 cups

[1]If the package directions call for whole or skim milk, the data given here are for whole milk unless otherwise stated.

FOOD/ DESCRIPTION	MEASURE OR QUANTITY	FATS IN GRAMS		
		Total	Saturated	Unsaturated
ABALONE (USDA) canned	4 oz.	.3		
AC'CENT	¼ tsp. (1 gram)	0.0		
AGNOLETTI, frozen (Buitoni):				
Cheese filled	2 oz.	3.3		
Meat filled	2 oz.	4.8		
ALBACORE, raw, meat only (USDA)	4 oz.	8.6	3.0	5.0
ALMOND:				
In shell (USDA)	4 oz. (weighed in shell)	31.4	2.0	29.0
Shelled:				
Plain, unsalted, whole (USDA)	1 oz.	15.4	1.0	14.0
Blanched, salted (USDA)	1 cup (5.5 oz.)	90.6	8.0	83.0
Chocolate-covered (See **CANDY**)				
Roasted, salted:				
(USDA)	1 oz.	16.4	1.0	15.0
(Eagle) *Honey Roast*	1 oz.	12.0		
(Planters) dry roasted or smoked	1 oz.	15.0		
ALMOND BUTTER (Hain) raw or toasted	1 T.	9.5	1.0	2.0
ALMOND DELIGHT, cereal (Ralston-Purina)	¾ cup (1 oz.)	2.0		
ALPHA-BITS, cereal (Post)	1 cup (1 oz.)	1.1		
ANCHOVY PASTE, canned (Grandaisa)	½ of 2-oz. can	2.5		
ANCHOVY, PICKLED, canned (Grandaisa)	1 oz.	2.5		
ANGEL FOOD CAKE (See **CAKE,** Angel Food)				
APPLE, any variety:				
Fresh (USDA):				
With skin	1 med., 2½" dia. (about 3 per lb.)	.8		
Without skin	1 med., 2½" dia. (about 3 per lb.)	.4		
Pared, quartered	1 cup (4.3 oz.)	.4		
Canned (See also **APPLE-SAUCE**):				
(Comstock) rings	1.1-oz. piece	.5		
(White House):				
Rings, spiced	.5-oz. ring	0.0		
Sliced	½ cup (4 oz.)	0.0		
Dehydrated:				
Uncooked (USDA)	1 oz.	.6		
Cooked, sweetened (USDA)	½ cup (4.2 oz.)	.4		
(Weight Watchers):				
Chips	¾-oz. pouch	0.0		
Snacks	.5-oz. pouch	<1.0		
Dried:				
Uncooked (USDA)	1 cup (3 oz.)	1.4		
Cooked (USDA) sweetened or unsweetened	½ cup	.6		
Frozen, sweetened, sliced, not thawed (USDA)	4 oz.	.1		
APPLE BROWN BETTY, home recipe (USDA)	1 cup (8.1 oz.)	8.0	2.0	6.0
APPLE BUTTER (Home Brands)	1 T. (.7 oz.)	0.0		
APPLE CHERRY JUICE, canned (Red Cheek)	6 fl. oz.	0.0		
APPLE-CRANBERRY JUICE DRINK:				
Canned (Mott's)	8.45-fl.-oz. cont.	0.0		
*Frozen (Tree Top)	6 fl. oz.	0.0		
APPLE DRINK:				
Canned:				
(Johanna Farms) *Ssips*	½ cup	0.0		
(Mott's) sweet	½ cup	0.0		
*Mix (Country Time)	8 fl. oz.	0.0		

FOOD DESCRIPTION	MEASURE OR QUANTITY	FATS IN GRAMS		
		Total	Saturated	Unsaturated
APPLE DUMPLING, frozen				
(Pepperidge Farm)	1 dumpling (3.3 oz.)	16.4		
APPLE, ESCALLOPED:				
Canned (White House)	½ cup (4.5 oz.)	1.0		
Frozen (Stouffer's)	4-oz. serving	2.0		
APPLE-GRAPE JUICE, canned				
(Mott's) or (Tree Top)	6 fl. oz.	0.0		
APPLE JACKS, cereal				
(Kellogg's)	1 cup (1 oz.)	0.0		
APPLE JELLY	Any quantity	0.0		
APPLE JUICE:				
Canned:				
(Borden's) *Sippin' Pak*	8.45 fl.-oz. cont.	0.0		
(Johanna Farms) Florida citrus or *Tree-Ripe*	8.45-fl.-oz. cont.	Tr.		
(Land O'Lakes)	6 fl. oz.	0.0		
(Mott's)	6 fl. oz.	0.0		
(Red Cheek)	6 fl. oz.	0.0		
Chilled (Minute Maid)	6 fl. oz.	.2		
*Frozen (Minute Maid)	6 fl. oz.	Tr.		
APPLE JUICE DRINK, canned				
(General Mills) *Squeezit*	6¾-oz.	< 1.0		
APPLE NECTAR, canned				
(Libby's)	6 fl. oz.	0.0		
APPLE-PEAR JUICE, canned				
or *frozen (Tree Top)	6 fl. oz.	0.0		
APPLE PIE (See **PIE,** Apple)				
APPLE RAISIN CRISP, cereal				
(Kellogg's)	⅔ cup (1.3 oz.)	0.0		
APPLESAUCE, canned:				
Sweetened (Mott's) any type	6 oz.	0.0		
Unsweetened, dietetic or low-calorie:				
(USDA)	½ cup (4.3 oz.)	.2		
(White House) regular or with apple juice added	½ cup	0.0		
APPLE STRUDEL, frozen				
(Pepperidge Farm)	3-oz. serving	11.0		
APRICOT:				
Fresh (USDA):				
Whole	1 lb. (weighed with pits)	.9		
Halves	1 cup (5.5 oz.)	.3		
Canned, regular pack, solids & liq.:				
Juice pack (USDA)	4 oz.	.2		
Light syrup (USDA)	4 oz.	.1		
Heavy syrup:				
Halves & syrup (USDA)	½ cup (4.4 oz.)	.1		
Halves & syrup (USDA)	4 med. halves with 2 T. syrup (4.3 oz.)	.1		
(Del Monte)	½ cup (4.4 oz.)	0.0		
Canned, unsweetened or low-calorie:				
(Diet Delight)	½ cup (4.4 oz.)	< .1		
(Libby's)	½ cup (4.4 oz.)	0.0		
Dehydrated (USDA):				
Uncooked	4 oz.	1.1		
Cooked, sugar added, solids & liq.	4 oz.	.2		
Dried:				
Uncooked:				
(USDA)	1 lb.	2.3		
(USDA)	½ cup (2.3 oz.)	.3		
(Del Monte)	½ cup (2.3 oz.)	0.0		
Cooked (USDA) sweetened or unsweetened	½ cup with liq.	.2		
Frozen, sweetened, not thawed (USDA)	4 oz.	.1		
APRICOT, CANDIED (USDA)	1 oz.	< .1		

FOOD DESCRIPTION	MEASURE OR QUANTITY	Total	Saturated	Unsaturated
APRICOT LIQUEUR (Leroux) 60 proof	1 oz.	0.0		
APRICOT NECTAR, canned, sweetened (Ardmore Farms)	6 fl. oz.	Tr.		
APRICOT & PINEAPPLE PRESERVE:				
Sweetened (Bama)	1 T. (.7 oz.)	< .1		
Dietetic or low-calorie (Diet Delight)	1 T. (.6 oz.)	0.0		
APRICOT PRESERVE:				
Sweetened (Home Brand)	1 T.	0.0		
Dietetic or low-calorie (Estee)	1 T. (.6 oz.)	0.0		
ARBY'S:				
Bac'n Cheddar Deluxe	7.85-oz. serving	34.0		
Chicken breast sandwich	7¼-oz. serving	27.0		
Croissant:				
Bacon & egg	4½-oz. serving	25.0		
Butter	2-oz. serving	10.0		
Chicken salad	5-oz. serving	36.0		
Ham & swiss	4-oz. serving	15.0		
Sausage & egg	5¾-oz. serving	35.0		
French fries	2½-oz. serving	8.0		
Ham & cheese, hot	1 serving	13.0		
Potato cake	3-oz. serving	14.0		
Potato, super stuffed:				
Broccoli & cheddar	12-oz. serving	22.0		
Deluxe	11.1-oz. serving	38.0		
Mushroom & cheese	10½-oz. serving	22.0		
Taco	15-oz. serving	27.0		
Roast beef:				
Regular	5.2-oz. serving	15.0		
Junior	3-oz. serving	8.0		
King	6.7-oz. serving	19.0		
Super	8.3-oz. serving	22.0		
Shake:				
Chocolate	10.6-oz. serving	11.0		
Vanilla	8.8-oz. serving	10.0		
Turkey, deluxe, sandwich	7-oz. serving	17.0		
ARTICHOKE, Globe or French (See also **JERUSALEM ARTICHOKE**):				
Raw, whole (USDA)	1 lb. (weighed untrimmed)	.4		
Boiled, without salt, drained (USDA)	4 oz.	.2		
Frozen (Birds Eye) hearts	5–6 hearts (3 oz.)	.4		
ASPARAGUS:				
Raw, whole spears (USDA)	1 lb. (weighed untrimmed)	.5		
Boiled, without salt, whole spears (USDA)	4 spears (½" dia. at base, 2.1 oz.)	.1		
Canned, regular pack, green or white: (USDA):				
Spears & liq.	4 oz.	.3		
Spears only	6 med. spears (3.4 oz.)	.4		
(Green Giant) solids & liq., cuts	½ of 8-oz. can	0.0		
Canned, dietetic pack, green or white:				
(Diet Delight) solids & liq.	½ cup (4.2 oz.)	0.0		
(S&W) *Nutradiet,* spears, green label, solids & liq.	½ cup	0.0		
Frozen:				
(Birds Eye) cuts or spears	⅓ of 10-oz. pkg.	0.0		
(McKenzie) spears	3⅓ oz.	0.0		
ASPARAGUS PILAF, frozen (Green Giant) microwave garden gourmet	9½-oz. pkg.	4.0	2.0	2.0

FOOD DESCRIPTION	MEASURE OR QUANTITY	FATS IN GRAMS		
		Total	Saturated	Unsaturated
AUNT JEMIMA SYRUP (See **SYRUP,** Pancake or Waffle)				
AVOCADO, PEELED, PITTED (USDA):				
All commercial varieties:				
Whole	1 lb. (weighed with seed & skin)	55.8	11.0	45.0
Diced	½ cup (2.6 oz.)	12.1	2.0	10.0
California varieties, mainly Fuerte:				
Whole	½ avocado (3⅛" dia.)	18.4	3.0	15.0
½" cubes	½ cup (2.7 oz.)	12.9	2.0	11.0
AVOCADO PUREE (Calavo)	½ cup (8.1 oz.)	36.4	5.6	30.5
***AWAKE** (Birds Eye)	½ cup (4.4 oz.)	.3		
BACON, cured:				
Raw (USDA):				
Sliced	1 lb.	314.3	101.0	213.0
Slab	1 lb. (weighed with rind)	295.5	95.0	200.0
Broiled or fried, crisp, drained:				
(USDA) thin slice	1 slice (5 grams)	2.6	<1.0	2.0
(USDA) thick slice	1 slice (.4 oz.)	6.2	2.0	4.0
(Oscar Mayer):				
Regular	6-gram slice	3.1	1.2	1.9
Lower salt	6.1-gram slice	2.6	.9	1.6
Canned (USDA)	3 oz.	60.8	20.0	41.0
BACON BITS:				
Real (Oscar Mayer)	1 tsp (.1 oz.)	.3	.1	.2
Imitation (Durkee)	1 tsp.	.4		
BACON, CANADIAN:				
Unheated:				
(USDA)	1 oz.	4.1	1.0	3.0
(Oscar Mayer)	.85-oz. slice	.8	.3	.4
Broiled or fried, drained (USDA)	1 oz.	5.0	2.0	3.0
BACON, SIMULATED, COOKED:				
(Oscar Mayer) *Lean 'N Tasty:*				
Beef	12-gram strip	3.9	1.5	2.2
Pork	13-gram strip	4.6	1.6	2.6
(Swift) *Sizzlean,* pork	.4-oz. strip	4.2		
BAKING POWDER, regular or low-sodium (USDA) phosphate, SAS or tartrate	1 tsp.	Tr.		
BAMBOO SHOOT:				
Raw (USDA) trimmed	4 oz.	.3		
Canned, drained solids (Chun King)	8½-oz. can	.7		
BANANA (USDA):				
Common:				
Fresh:				
Whole	1 lb. (weighed with skin)	.6		
Small size	4.9-oz. banana (7¾" × 1 11/32")	.2		
Large size	7-oz. banana	.3		
Chunks or sliced	1 cup (5 oz.)	.3		
Dehydrated, flakes	½ cup (1.8 oz.)	.4		
Red, fresh, whole	1 lb. (weighed with skin)	.6		
BANANA, BAKING (See **PLANTAIN**)				
BANANA NECTAR, canned (Libby's)	6 fl. oz.	0.0		
BANANA PIE, cream or custard (See **PIE,** banana)				
BARBECUE SEASONING (French's)	1 tsp. (2 grams)	Tr.		
BARLEY, pearled, dry:				
Light (Quaker Scotch)	¼ cup (1.7 oz.)	.5		
Pot or Scotch (USDA)	2 oz.	.6		

FOOD DESCRIPTION	MEASURE OR QUANTITY	FATS IN GRAMS		
		Total	Saturated	Unsaturated
BARRACUDA, raw, meat only (USDA)	4 oz.	2.9		
BASS (USDA):				
Black sea, raw, whole	1 lb. (weighed whole)	2.1		
Smallmouth & largemouth, raw, whole	1 lb. (weighed whole)	3.7		
Striped, raw, meat only	4 oz.	3.1		
White, raw, meat only	4 oz.	2.6		
BATMAN, cereal (Ralston-Purina)	1 cup (1 oz.)	1.0		
BEAN, BAKED, canned:				
(USDA):				
With pork & molasses sauce	1 cup (9 oz.)	12.0	5.0	7.0
With pork & tomato sauce	1 cup (9 oz.)	6.6	3.0	4.0
With tomato sauce	1 cup (9 oz.)	1.3		
(B&M) Brick Oven:				
Barbecue	7/8 cup (8 oz.)	6.0		
Honey	7/8 cup (8 oz.)	2.0		
Pea bean, small, in pork & molasses sauce or vegetarian	7/8 cup (8 oz.)	7.0		
In tomato sauce	7/8 cup (8 oz.)	3.0		
(Campbell):				
Home style	8 oz.	4.0		
Old-fashioned, in molasses & brown-sugar sauce	8 oz.	3.0		
(Grandma Brown's) home baked	8 oz.	1.7		
(Hunt's) & pork	8 oz.	2.0		
BEAN, BAYO, dry (USDA)	4 oz.	1.7		
BEAN, BLACK:				
Dry (USDA)	4 oz.	1.7		
Canned (Progresso)	1 cup	<2.0		
BEAN, BROWN, dry (USDA)	4 oz.	1.7		
BEAN, CALICO, dry (USDA)	4 oz.	1.4		
BEAN, CANNOLLINI, canned (Progresso)	1/2 cup	<1.0		
BEAN, FAVA, canned (Progresso)	1/2 cup	<1.0		
BEAN & FRANKFURTER, canned:				
(Campbell's) in tomato & molasses sauce	7⅞-oz. serving	14.0		
(Hormel) *Short Orders*	7½-oz. can	14.0		
BEAN & FRANKFURTER DINNER, frozen:				
(Banquet)	10-oz. dinner	25.0		
(Morton)	10-oz. dinner	13.0		
BEAN, GARBANZO, canned, solids & liq. (Old El Paso)	1/2 cup	<1.0		
BEAN, GREEN OR SNAP:				
Fresh (USDA):				
Whole	1 lb. (weighed untrimmed)	.8		
1½″ to 2″ pieces	1/2 cup (1.8 oz.)	.1		
French-style	1/2 cup (1.4 oz.)	<.1		
Boiled without salt, drained, whole or pieces (USDA)	1/2 cup (2.2 oz.)	.1		
Canned, regular pack:				
(Allen) solids & liq.	1/2 cup	0.0		
(Larsen) *Freshlike*, solids & liq.	1/2 cup	0.0		
Canned, dietetic pack:				
(USDA)	4 oz.	.1		
(Del Monte) solids & liq.	1/2 cup (4.2 oz.)	0.0		
Frozen:				
(Birds Eye):				
Cut:				
Plain	1/4 of 12-oz. pkg.	.1		
With mushrooms	5-oz. serving	2.7		

FOOD DESCRIPTION	MEASURE OR QUANTITY	FATS IN GRAMS		
		Total	Saturated	Unsaturated
French cut:				
Plain	⅓ of 9-oz. pkg.	Tr.		
With toasted almonds	⅓ of 9-oz. pkg.	1.6		
Whole	⅓ of 9-oz. pkg.	.2		
(Green Giant):				
In butter sauce:				
Regular	⅓ of 9-oz. pkg.	1.0	<1.0	0.0
One serving	5½-oz. pkg.	2.0	<2.0	0.0
Harvest Fresh, cut	⅓ of 8-oz. pkg.	0.0		
Polybag	½ cup (2.5 oz.)	0.0		
BEAN, GREEN, & MUSHROOM CASSEROLE, frozen (Stouffer's)	½ of 9½-oz. pkg.	11.0		
BEAN, KIDNEY OR RED:				
Dry (USDA)	4 oz.	1.7		
Cooked without salt (USDA)	½ cup (3.3 oz.)	.5		
Canned, solids & liq.:				
(Comstock)	½ cup (4.4 oz.)	0.0		
(Goya) red or white	½ cup	.5		
Dietetic (S&W) Nutradiet, green label, low-sodium	½ cup	.3		
BEAN, LIMA, young:				
Raw, without shell (USDA)	1 lb. (weighed shelled)	2.3		
Boiled without salt, drained (USDA)	½ cup (3 oz.)	.4		
Canned, regular pack:				
(USDA) solids & liq.	½ cup (4.4 oz.)	.4		
(Allen) solids & liq.	4 oz.	1.0		
(Comstock) solids & liq., regular or butter	½ cup (4.4 oz.)	0.0		
Canned, dietetic pack:				
(USDA) low-sodium, solids & liq. or drained solids	4 oz.	.3		
(Larsen) Fresh-Lite, water packed, solids & liq.	½ cup (4.4 oz.)	0.0		
Frozen:				
(Birds Eye):				
Baby limas	½ cup (3.3 oz.)	.5		
Fordhooks	⅓ of 10-oz. pkg.	.3		
(Green Giant):				
In butter sauce	⅓ of 10-oz. pkg.	3.6		
Harvest Fresh	⅓ of 9-oz. pkg.	0.0		
BEAN, LIMA, mature (USDA):				
Dry, baby or large	½ cup	1.4		
Boiled without salt, drained	½ cup (3.4 oz.)	.6		
BEAN, MUNG, dry (USDA)	½ cup (3.7 oz.)	1.4		
BEAN, PINK, canned (Goya)	½ cup	.5		
BEAN, PINTO:				
Dry (USDA)	4 oz.	1.4		
Canned:				
(Gebhardt)	½ of 15-oz. can	1.0		
(Goya)	½ cup (4 oz.)	.5		
BEAN, RED (See **BEAN, KIDNEY** or **BEAN, RED MEXICAN**)				
BEAN, RED MEXICAN:				
Dry (USDA)	4 oz.	1.4		
Canned:				
(Goya)	1 cup	.2		
(Old El Paso)	½ cup	1.0		
BEAN, REFRIED, canned, solids & liq.:				
(Gebhardt) regular or jalapeño	4 oz.	2.0		
(Old El Paso):				
With bacon	½ cup	8.0		
With cheese, jalapeños, spicy or vegetarian	½ cup	2.0		
With sausage	½ cup	16.0		

FOOD DESCRIPTION	MEASURE OR QUANTITY	FATS IN GRAMS		
		Total	Saturated	Unsaturated
(Rosarita):				
Regular, spicy or vegetarian	½ cup	2.0		
With green chilies or beans & onion	½ cup	1.9		
With nacho cheese & onion	½ cup	2.3		
BEAN, ROMAN, canned, solids & liq. (Goya)	½ cup (2.3 oz.)	.2		
BEAN SALAD, canned, solids & liq. (Green Giant)	½ cup	0.0		
BEANS 'N FIXIN'S, canned (Hunt's) *Big John's:*				
Beans	3 oz.	<1.0		
Fixin's	1 oz.	2.0		
BEAN SOUP (See **SOUP,** Bean)				
BEAN SPROUT:				
Ming:				
Raw (USDA)	½ lb.	.4		
Boiled without salt, drained (USDA)	½ cup (2.2 oz.)	.1		
Soy:				
Raw (USDA)	½ lb.	3.2		
Boiled without salt, drained (USDA)	½ cup (1.9 oz.)	.8		
Canned (La Choy) drained solids	⅔ cup	<1.0		
BEAN, WHITE, dry:				
Raw (USDA):				
Great Northern	½ cup (3.1 oz.)	1.4		
Navy or pea	½ cup (3.7 oz.)	1.7		
Cooked without salt (USDA):				
Great Northern	½ cup (3 oz.)	.5		
Navy or pea	½ cup (3.4 oz.)	.6		
BEAN, YELLOW OR WAX:				
Raw, whole (USDA)	1 lb. (weighed untrimmed)	.8		
Boiled without salt, drained (USDA)	4 oz.	.2		
Canned, regular pack:				
(USDA) solids & liq. or drained solids	½ cup (2.2 oz.)	.2		
(Larsen) *Freshlike,* cut, solids & liq.	½ cup (4.2 oz.)	0.0		
Canned, dietetic pack (Larsen) *Fresh-Lite,* water pack, solids & liq.	½ cup (4.2 oz.)	0.0		
Frozen (Larsen) cut	3 oz.	0.0		
BEAR CLAWS (Dolly Madison) chocolate or cinnamon	2¾-oz. piece	13.0		
BEECHNUT (USDA) shelled	1 oz. (weighed shelled)	14.2	1.0	13.0
BEEF. Values for beef cuts are given below for "lean and fat" and for "lean only." Beef purchased by the consumer at the retail store usually is trimmed to about one-half inch layer of fat. This is the meat described as "lean and fat." If all the fat that can be cut off with a knife is removed, the remainder is the "lean only." These cuts still contain flecks of fat known as "marbling" distributed through the meat. Cooked meats are medium done.				
Choice grade cuts (USDA):				
Brisket:				
Raw, lean & fat	1 lb. (weighed with bone)	112.4	54.0	58.0
Raw, lean & fat	1 lb. (weighed without bone)	133.8	64.0	69.0
Raw, lean only	1 lb.	37.2	18.0	20.0

FOOD DESCRIPTION	MEASURE OR QUANTITY	FATS IN GRAMS		
		Total	Saturated	Unsaturated
Braised:				
Lean & fat	4 oz.	39.5	19.0	21.0
Lean only	4 oz.	11.9	6.0	6.0
Chuck:				
Raw, lean & fat	1 lb. (weighed with bone)	75.0	36.0	39.0
Raw, lean & fat	1 lb. (weighed without bone)	88.9	43.0	46.0
Raw, lean only	1 lb.	33.6	18.0	15.0
Braised or pot-roasted:				
Lean & fat	4 oz.	27.1	13.0	14.0
Lean only	4 oz.	10.8	5.0	6.0
Dried (See BEEF, CHIPPED)				
Fat, separable, raw	1 oz.	21.6	10.0	11.0
Fat, separable, cooked	1 oz.	22.1	10.0	12.0
Filet Mignon. There is no data available on its composition. For dietary estimates, the data for sirloin steak, lean only, afford the closest approximation.				
Flank:				
Raw, 100% lean	1 lb.	25.9	12.0	13.0
Braised, 100% lean	4 oz.	8.3	4.0	4.0
Foreshank:				
Raw, lean & fat	1 lb. (weighed with bone)	34.8	17.0	18.0
Simmered:				
Lean & fat	4 oz.	19.4	9.0	10.0
Lean only	4 oz.	6.6	3.0	3.0
Ground:				
Regular:				
Raw	1 lb.	96.2	48.0	48.0
Raw	1 cup (8 oz.)	47.9	23.0	25.0
Broiled	4 oz.	23.0	11.0	12.
Lean:				
Raw	1 lb.	45.4	22.0	23.0
Raw	1 cup (8 oz.)	22.6	11.0	11.0
Broiled	4 oz.	12.8	6.0	7.0
Heel of round:				
Raw, lean & fat	1 lb.	64.4	31.0	34.0
Raw, lean only	1 lb.	21.3	9.0	12.0
Roasted:				
Lean & fat	4 oz.	18.3	9.0	10.0
Lean only	4 oz.	6.5	3.0	3.0
Hindshank:				
Raw:				
Lean & fat	1 lb. (weighed with bone)	48.9	23.0	25.0
Lean & fat	1 lb. (weighed without bone)	106.1	51.0	55.0
Lean only	1 lb.	20.9	10.0	11.0
Simmered:				
Lean & fat	4 oz.	31.9	15.0	17.0
Lean only	4 oz.	6.7	3.0	4.0
Neck:				
Raw, lean & fat	1 lb. (weighed with bone)	57.7	28.0	30.0
Pot-roasted:				
Lean & fat	4 oz.	22.3	11.0	12.0
Lean only	4 oz.	8.3	4.0	4.0
Oxtail, raw	1 lb. (weighed with bone)	7.9	4.0	4.0
Oxtail, raw	1 lb. (weighed without bone)	31.8	15.0	17.0
Plate:				
Raw:				
Lean & fat	1 lb. (weighed with bone)	150.6	72.0	78.0
Lean & fat	1 lb. (weighed without bone)	169.2	81.0	88.0
Lean only	1 lb.	37.2	18.0	20.0
Simmered:				
Lean & fat	4 oz.	48.5	23.0	25.0
Lean only	4 oz.	11.9	6.0	6.0
Rib roast:				
Raw:				
Lean & fat	1 lb. (weighed with bone)	156.1	75.0	81.0
Lean & fat	1 lb. (weighed without bone)	169.6	81.0	88.0
Lean only	1 lb.	52.6	27.0	25.0

FOOD DESCRIPTION	MEASURE OR QUANTITY	FATS IN GRAMS		
		Total	Saturated	Unsaturated
Roasted:				
Lean & fat	4 oz.	44.7	21.0	23.0
Lean only	4 oz.	15.2	7.0	8.0
Lean only, chopped	1 cup (4.5 oz.)	17.2	8.0	9.0
Lean only, diced	1 cup (5 oz.)	19.2	9.0	10.0
Round:				
Raw:				
Lean & fat	1 lb. (weighed with bone)	53.9	26.0	28.0
Lean & fat	1 lb. (weighed without bone)	55.8	27.0	29.0
Lean only	1 lb.	21.3	9.0	12.0
Broiled:				
Lean & fat	4 oz.	17.5	8.0	9.0
Lean only	4 oz.	6.9	3.0	4.0
Rump:				
Raw:				
Lean & fat	1 lb. (weighed with bone)	97.4	47.0	50.0
Lean & fat	1 lb. (weighed without bone)	114.8	55.0	60.0
Lean only	1 lb.	34.0	15.0	19.0
Roasted:				
Lean & fat	4 oz.	31.0	15.0	16.0
Lean only	4 oz.	10.5	5.0	5.0
Steak, club:				
Raw:				
Lean & fat	1 lb. (weighed with bone)	132.1	63.0	69.0
Lean & fat	1 lb. (weighed without bone)	157.9	76.0	82.0
Lean only	1 lb.	46.7	22.0	25.0
Broiled:				
Lean & fat	4 oz.	46.0	22.0	24.0
Lean only	4 oz.	14.7	7.0	8.0
One 8-oz. steak (weighed without bone before cooking) will give you:				
Lean & fat	5.9 oz.	67.4	32.0	35.0
Lean only	3.4 oz.	12.5	6.0	7.0
Steak, porterhouse:				
Raw, lean & fat	1 lb. (weighed with bone)	148.8	71.0	78.0
Broiled:				
Lean & fat	4 oz.	47.9	23.0	25.0
Lean only	4 oz.	11.9	6.0	6.0
One 16-oz. steak (weighed with bone before cooking) will give you:				
Lean & fat	10.2 oz.	121.5	59.0	63.0
Lean only	5.9 oz.	17.4	8.0	9.0
Steak, ribeye, broiled:				
One 10-oz. steak (weighed without bone before cooking) will give you:				
Lean & fat	7.3 oz.	81.6	39.0	42.0
Lean only	3.8 oz.	14.3	7.0	7.0
Steak, sirloin, double-bone:				
Raw:				
Lean & fat	1 lb. (weighed with bone)	108.4	52.0	56.0
Lean & fat	1 lb. (weighed without bone)	132.0	63.0	69.0
Lean only	1 lb.	33.6	18.0	15.0
Broiled:				
Lean & fat	4 oz.	39.3	19.0	20.0
Lean only	4 oz.	10.8	5.0	6.0
One 16-oz. steak (weighed with bone before cooking) will give you:				
Lean & fat	8.9 oz.	87.4	42.0	45.0
Lean only	5.9 oz.	15.8	8.0	8.0
One 12-oz. steak (weighed with bone before cooking) will give you:				
Lean & fat	6.6 oz.	65.2	31.0	34.0
Lean only	4.4 oz.	11.8	6.0	6.0

FOOD DESCRIPTION	MEASURE OR QUANTITY	FATS IN GRAMS		
		Total	**Saturated**	**Unsaturated**
Steak, sirloin, hipbone:				
Raw:				
Lean & fat	1 lb. (weighed with bone)	149.3	72.0	78.0
Lean & fat	1 lb. (weighed without bone)	176.0	84.0	92.0
Lean only	1 lb.	44.9	21.0	24.0
Broiled:				
Lean & fat	4 oz.	50.9	24.0	26.0
Lean only	4 oz.	14.2	7.0	7.0
Steak, sirloin, wedge & round-bone:				
Raw:				
Lean & fat	1 lb. (weighed with bone)	112.3	54.0	58.0
Lean & fat	1 lb. (weighed without bone)	121.1	58.0	63.0
Lean only	1 lb.	25.9	12.0	14.0
Broiled:				
Lean & fat	4 oz.	36.3	17.0	19.0
Lean only	4 oz.	8.7	4.0	5.0
Steak, T-bone:				
Raw, lean & fat	1 lb. (weighed with bone)	149.1	72.0	78.0
Broiled:				
Lean & fat	4 oz.	49.0	24.0	26.0
Lean only	4 oz.	11.7	6.0	6.0
One 16-oz. steak (weighed with bone before cooking) will give you:				
Lean & fat	9.8 oz.	120.1	58.0	63.0
Lean only	5.5 oz.	16.1	8.0	8.0
BEEFAMATO, cocktail, canned (Mott's)	6 fl. oz.	0.0		
BEEF BOUILLON/BROTH, cubes or powder (See also **SOUP,** Beef):				
(Herb-Ox)	1 cube or 1 packet	.1		
*(Knorr)	8 fl. oz.	1.1		
BEEF, CHIPPED:				
Uncooked. (USDA)	½ cup (2.9 oz.)	5.2	2.0	3.0
Cooked, creamed, home recipe (USDA)	1 cup (8.6 oz.)	25.2	15.0	11.0
Frozen, creamed:				
(Banquet)	4-oz. pkg.	25.2	15.0	11.0
(Stouffer's)	5.5-oz. serving	16.0		
BEEF DINNER OR ENTREE:				
*Canned (Hunt's) Entree Maker	7.6-oz. serving	12.0		
Frozen:				
(Armour):				
Classic Lite, Steak Diane	10-oz. pkg.	9.0		
Dining Lite, teriyaki	9-oz. pkg.	5.0		
Dinner Classics:				
Sirloin roast	10.4-oz. pkg.	4.0		
Sirloin tips	10¼-oz. pkg.	7.0		
(Banquet):				
Chopped	11-oz. pkg.	32.0		
Extra Helping	16-oz. pkg.	61.0		
(Healthy Choice) sirloin tips	11¾-oz. pkg.	6.0	3.0	< 1.0
(La Choy) Fresh & Light, & broccoli with rice	11-oz. pkg.	5.0		
(Stouffer's):				
Lean Cuisine:				
Oriental, with vegetables & rice	8⅝-oz. pkg.	7.0		
Szechuan, with noodles & vegetables	9¼-oz. pkg.	10.0		
Right Course:				
Dijon	9½-oz. pkg.	9.0		
Fiesta	8⅞-oz. pkg.	7.0		
(Swanson):				
4-compartment dinner:				
Regular	11½-oz. dinner	8.0		
Chopped sirloin	11½-oz. dinner	17.0		

FOOD DESCRIPTION	MEASURE OR QUANTITY	FATS IN GRAMS		
		Total	Saturated	Unsaturated
Hungry-Man:				
Chopped	17¼-oz. meal	19.0		
Sliced	16-oz. pkg.	12.0		
(Weight Watchers):				
London broil in mushroom sauce	7.37-oz. pkg.	3.0	1.0	2.0
Sirloin tips & mushrooms in wine sauce	7.5-oz. pkg.	8.0	4.0	4.0
BEEF, DRIED, packaged (Hormel) sliced	1 oz.	1.0		
*****BEEF, GROUND, SEASONING MIX** (Durkee) plain or with onion	1 cup	48.5		
BEEF HASH, ROAST, frozen (Stouffer's)	10-oz. pkg.	22.0		
BEEF, PACKAGED (Carl Buddig)	1 oz.	2.0	1.0	Tr.
BEEF PEPPER ORIENTAL:				
Canned (La Choy)	¾ cup	2.0		
Frozen (La Choy)	12-oz. pkg.	3.0		
BEEF PIE:				
Baked, home recipe (USDA)	⅓ of 9″ pie (7.4 oz.)	30.4	8.0	22.0
Frozen:				
(Empire Kosher)	8-oz. pie	30.0		
(Morton)	7-oz. pie	31.0		
(Swanson):				
Regular	8-oz. pie	21.0		
Hungry-Man, regular	16-oz. pie	34.0		
BEEF, POTTED (USDA)	1 oz.	5.4		
BEEF RIBS, frozen:				
(Armour) *Dinner Classics,* boneless	9¾-oz. pkg.	16.0		
(Stouffer's) boneless, with gravy	9-oz. pkg.	20.0		
BEEF SOUP (See **SOUP,** Beef)				
BEEF SPREAD, ROAST, canned (Underwood)	½ of 4¾-oz. can	10.0		
BEEF STEW:				
Home recipe, made with lean beef chuck (USDA)	1 cup (8.6 oz.)	10.5	5.0	6.0
Canned:				
Regular:				
(USDA)	1 cup (8.6 oz.)	7.6		
Dinty Moore:				
Regular	½ of 24-oz. can	12.0		
Short Orders	7½-oz. serving	9.0		
(Libby's)	½ of 24-oz. can	6.0		
Dietetic (Estee)	7½-oz. serving	11.0		
Frozen (Banquet) *Family Entrees*	¼ of 28.2-oz. pkg.	5.0		
*****BEEF STEW SEASONING MIX** (Durkee)	1 cup	24.0		
*****BEEF STROGANOFF SEASONING MIX** (Durkee)	1 cup	71.1		
BEER, canned	Any quantity	0.0		
BEET:				
Raw, diced (USDA)	½ cup (2.4 oz.)	< 1.0		
Boiled (USDA) whole, drained	2 beets (2″ dia., 3.5 oz.)	.1		
Canned, regular pack:				
(Comstock) regular or pickled, solids & liq.	½ cup (4.2 oz.)	0.0		
(Larsen) *Freshlike,* pickled, sliced or whole	½ cup	0.0		
Canned, dietetic pack:				
(Del Monte) sliced, low-salt, solids & liq.	½ cup (4 oz.)	0.0		
(Larsen) *Fresh-Lite,* sliced, solids & liq.	½ cup (4.3 oz.)	0.0		

FOOD DESCRIPTION	MEASURE OR QUANTITY	FATS IN GRAMS		
		Total	Saturated	Unsaturated
BEET GREENS (USDA):				
Raw, whole	1 lb. (weighed untrimmed)	.8		
Boiled, leaves & stems, drained	½ cup (2.6 oz.)	.1		
BERRY BEARS (General Mills), *Fruit Corners*	.9-oz. pouch	< 1.0		
BERRY, MIXED, DRINK:				
Canned (Johanna Farms) *Ssips*	8.45 fl. oz.	0.0		
*Mix, dietetic, *Crystal Light*	8 fl. oz.	0.0		
BIGG MIXX, cereal (Kellogg's), plain or with raisins	½ cup	2.0		
BIG MAC (See **McDONALD'S**)				
BISCUIT (USDA) baking powder, home recipe, made with regular flour & lard or vegetable shortening	1-oz. biscuit (2" dia.)	4.8		
BISCUIT DOUGH:				
Frozen, commercial (USDA)	1 oz.	3.4	< 1.0	2.0
Refrigerated:				
(USDA) commercial (Pillsbury):	1 oz.	3.4	< 1.0	< 2.0
Baking powder, *1869 Brand*	1 piece	5.0	1.0	< 1.0
Buttermilk:				
Regular	1 piece	1.0	Tr.	0.0
Ballard Oven Ready	1 piece	1.0	Tr.	0.0
Big Country	1 piece	4.0	1.0	0.0
Hungry Jack:				
Extra rich	1 piece	1.0	< 1.0	0.0
Flaky or fluffy	1 piece	4.0	1.0	0.0
Butter Tastin':				
Big Country	1 piece	4.0	1.0	0.0
1869 Brand	1 piece	5.0	1.0	< 1.0
Flaky, *Hungry Jack:*				
Regular or honey	1 piece	4.0	1.0	0.0
Butter Tastin'	1 piece	4.0	2.0	0.0
Heat'n Eat, Big Premium	1 piece	7.5	1.5	< 1.0
Oven Ready, Ballard	1 piece	1.0	0.0	0.0
BISCUIT MIX (USDA):				
Dry, with enriched flour	1 oz.	3.6	< 1.0	3.0
Baked from mix, with added milk	1-oz. biscuit	2.6	< 1.0	2.0
BLACKBERRY (USDA):				
Fresh (includes boysenberry, dewberry, youngberry, hulled	½ cup (2.6 oz.)	.7		
Canned, regular pack, solids & liq.:				
Juice pack	4 oz.	.9		
Heavy syrup	½ cup (4.6 oz.)	.8		
Canned, water pack, solids & liq.	½ cup (4.3 oz.)	.7		
Frozen, sweetened or unsweetened	4 oz.	.3		
BLACKBERRY JELLY				
(Smucker's) sweetened or dietetic	1 T.	0.0		
BLACKBERRY PRESERVE OR JAM:				
Sweetened (Home Brand)	1 T. (.7 oz.)	0.0		
Low-calorie (Estee)	1 T. (.6 oz.)	0.0		
BLACK-EYED PEA:				
Canned, regular pack, solids & liq.:				
(Allen):				
Regular	½ cup (4 oz.)	0.0		
With snap peas	½ cup (4 oz.)	2.0		
(Goya)	½ cup (4 oz.)	0.0		

FOOD DESCRIPTION	MEASURE OR QUANTITY	FATS IN GRAMS		
		Total	Saturated	Unsaturated
Frozen:				
(Birds Eye)	1/3 of 10-oz. pkg.	.6		
(Larsen)	3.3 oz.	.1		
BLINTZ, frozen:				
(Empire Kosher Foods):				
Apple, blueberry, cherry or cheese	2½-oz. piece	1.0		
Potato	2½-oz. piece	4.0		
(King Kold) cheese	2½-oz. piece	1.9		
BLOOD PUDDING OR SAUSAGE (USDA)	1 oz.	10.5	4.0	7.0
BLOODY MARY MIX (Holland House) liquid	1 fl. oz.	0.0		
BLUEBERRY (USDA):				
Fresh, trimmed	½ cup (2.6 oz.)	.4		
Canned, solids & liq:				
Syrup pack, extra heavy, or water pack	½ cup (4.3 oz.)	.2		
Frozen, solids & liq., sweetened or unsweetened	½ cup	.4		
BLUEBERRY PIE (See **PIE,** Blueberry)				
BLUEBERRY PRESERVE OR JAM:				
Sweetened (Home Brand)	1 T.	0.0		
Dietetic (Estee)	1 T. (.6 oz.)	0.0		
BLUEFISH (USDA):				
Raw, meat only	4 oz.	3.7		
Baked or broiled	4.4-oz. piece (3½″ × 3″ × ½″)	6.5		
Fried	5.3-oz. piece (3½″ × 3″ × ½″)	14.7		
BODY BUDDIES, cereal (General Mills) natural fruit flavor	1 cup (1 oz.)	1.0		
BOLOGNA:				
(USDA):				
All meat or with cereal	1 oz.	6.5		
(Eckrich):				
Beef:				
Regular	1-oz. slice	8.0		
Smorgas-Pac	¾-oz. slice	6.0		
Thick sliced	1½-oz. slice	12.0		
Garlic	1-oz. slice	8.0		
German brand, club or sliced	1-oz. serving	7.0		
Meat:				
Regular	1-oz. slice	8.0		
Thick sliced	1.7-oz. slice	14.0		
Hebrew National	1 oz.	8.0		
(Hormel):				
Beef:				
Regular	1 slice	8.0		
Ring, coarse ground	1 oz.	7.0		
Meat, regular	1 slice	8.0		
(Ohse):				
Beef	1 oz.	8.0		
Chicken, 15%	1 oz.	8.0		
Chicken, beef & pork	1 oz.	4.1	1.8	2.3
(Oscar Mayer):				
Beef	1-oz. slice	8.3	3.7	4.7
Garlic Beef	1-oz. slice	8.3	3.7	4.7
Meat	1-oz. slice	8.3	3.2	5.0
BOLOGNA & CHEESE:				
(Eckrich)	.7-oz. slice	8.0		
(Oscar Mayer)	.8-oz. slice	6.8	2.6	3.9
BONITO, raw (USDA) meat only	4 oz.	8.3		
BOO BERRY, cereal (General Mills)	1 cup (1 oz.)	1.0		

FOOD DESCRIPTION	MEASURE OR QUANTITY	FATS IN GRAMS		
		Total	Saturated	Unsaturated
BORSCHT, canned (Mother's) regular or dietetic	8 fl. oz.	.2		
BOSTON BROWN BREAD (see **BREAD**)				
BOSTON CREAM PIE (See **PIE,** Boston cream)				
BOUILLON CUBE (See also individual flavors) (USDA) flavor not indicated	1 cube (approx. ½", 4 grams)	.1		
BOURBON WHISKEY (See **DISTILLED LIQUOR**)				
BOYSENBERRY:				
Fresh (See **BLACKBERRY,** fresh)				
Canned, unsweetened or low-calorie water pack, solids & liq. (USDA)	4 oz.	.1		
Frozen, not thawed (USDA) sweetened or unsweetened	4 oz.	.3		
BOYSENBERRY JUICE, canned (Smucker's)	8 fl. oz.	0.0		
BOYSENBERRY PRESERVE OR JAM, low-calorie (S&W) *Nutradiet*	1 T. (.5 oz.)	< .1		
BRAINS, all animals, raw (USDA)	4 oz.	9.8		
BRAN (USDA):				
Crude	1 oz.	1.3		
With added sugar & defatted wheat germ	1 oz.	.5		
BRAN BREAKFAST CEREAL:				
(General Mills) *Raisin Nut Bran*	½ cup (1 oz.)	3.0		
(Kellogg's):				
All-Bran:				
Regular	⅓ cup (1 oz.)	1.0		
With extra fiber	½ cup (1 oz.)	0.0		
Bran Buds	⅓ cup (1 oz.)	1.0		
Oat:				
Common Sense, plain or raisin	½ cup	1.0		
Cracklin' Bran	½ cup (1 oz.)	4.0		
Raisin	¾ cup (1.4 oz.)	1.0		
(Malt-O-Meal):				
40% flakes	⅔ cup (1 oz.)	.9		
Raisin	¾ cup (1.4 oz.)	1.7		
(Post) flakes, natural	⅔ cup (1 oz.)	Tr.		
(Ralston-Purina):				
Bran News, apple or cinnamon	¾ cup (1 oz.)	0.0		
Chex	⅔ cup (1 oz.)	0.0		
BRANDY (See **DISTILLED LIQUOR**)				
BRAUNSCHWEIGER:				
(USDA)	2 slices (2" × ¼", .7 oz.)	5.5	2.0	4.0
(Oscar Mayer) chub or sliced	1 oz.	8.7	3.2	5.5
BRAZIL NUT (USDA) shelled	½ cup (2.5 oz.)	46.8	9.0	38.0
BREAD (listed by type or brand name; toasting does not affect these nutritive values, only weight):				
Boston brown (USDA)	1.7-oz. slice (3" × ¾")	120.0	.6	
Apple Cinnamon, *Pritikin*	1-oz. slice	1.0		
Bran (Roman Meal):				
5-Bran	1-oz. slice	1.1	.1	
Rice, honey or honey nut	1-oz. slice	1.8	.1	
Bran'nola (Arnold)	1.3-oz. slice	1.0		
Buttermilk, *Dutch Hearth*	1-oz. slice	2.0		
Buttertop, *Eddy's*	1-oz. slice	1.0		

FOOD DESCRIPTION	MEASURE OR QUANTITY	FATS IN GRAMS		
		Total	Saturated	Unsaturated
Cornbread (See **CORNBREAD**)				
Cracked-wheat:				
(Pepperidge Farm)	.9-oz. slice	1.0		
(Roman Meal)	1-oz. slice	.9	.1	
Egg, *Millbrook*	1-oz. slice	1.0		
Flatbread, *Ideal*	1 slice	Tr.		
French:				
(Arnold) *Francisco,* regular or international	1/16 of loaf (1 oz.)	1.0		
Eddy's, regular or sourdough	1-oz. slice	1.0		
Garlic (Arnold)	1-oz. slice	3.0		
Hi Fiber (Monks')	1-oz. slice	1.0		
Hollywood:				
Dark	1-oz. slice	1.1		
Light	1-oz. slice	.9		
Honey wheatberry:				
(Arnold)	1.1-oz. slice	2.0		
(Pepperidge Farm)	.9-oz. slice	1.0		
Italian:				
(Arnold) *Francisco*	1 slice	1.0		
Millbrook	1-oz. slice	1.0		
Low-sodium, *Eddy's*	1-oz. slice	2.0		
Multi-grain:				
Pritikin	1-oz. slice	1.0		
(Weight Watchers)	3/4-oz. slice	.6	Tr.	
Oat (Arnold), *Bran'nola,* country	1.3-oz. slice	1.0		
Oat bran (Roman Meal):				
Honey	1-oz. slice	1.1	.2	
Honey nut	1-oz. slice	1.6	.2	
Olympic meal, *Holsum*	1-oz. slice	1.0		
Onion dill, *Pritikin*	1-oz. slice	1.0		
Pumpernickel:				
(Levy's)	1.1-oz. slice	1.0		
(Pepperidge Farm):				
Family	1-oz. slice	1.0		
Party	6-gram slice	.2		
Raisin:				
(Monk's) cinnamon	1-oz. slice	2.0		
Pritikin	1-oz. slice	1.0		
(Weight Watchers)	.8-oz. slice	.6	Tr.	
Round top (Roman Meal) original	1-oz. slice	.9	Tr.	
Rye:				
(Arnold):				
Dill, with seeds or Jewish, with or without seeds	1.1-oz. slice	1.0		<.5
Melba thin	.7-oz. slice	.5		
(Levy's) real	1.1-oz. slice	1.0		
Pritikin	1-oz. slice	1.0		
(Weight Watchers)	3/4-oz. slice	.5	Tr.	
Sahara (Thomas'):				
White:				
Regular	2-oz. piece	1.0		
Large	3-oz. piece	2.0		
Whole wheat:				
Regular	2-oz. piece	2.0		
Mini	1-oz. piece	1.0		
Sandwich (Roman Meal)	.8-oz. slice	.9	Tr.	
7-Grain:				
Better Way	1-oz. slice	1.0		
(Roman Meal):				
Regular	1-oz. slice	.7	.1	
Light	.8-oz. slice	.4	Tr.	
Split Top, *Merita*	1-oz. slice	1.0		
Sunflower bran (Monk's)	1-oz. slice	1.0		
Toaster cake (See **TOASTER CAKE**)				

FOOD DESCRIPTION	MEASURE OR QUANTITY	FATS IN GRAMS		
		Total	Saturated	Unsaturated
Wheat:				
America's Own, cottage	1-oz. slice	1.0		
(Arnold):				
Bran'nola:				
Dark	1.3-oz. slice	1.0		
Hearty	1.3-oz. slice	2.0		
Brick Oven	1 slice	2.0		
Country	1.3-oz. slice	1.0		
Less	.8-oz. slice	0.0		
(Roman Meal) light	.8-oz. slice	.3	Tr.	
Wheatberry:				
Country Farms, honey	1½-oz. slice	2.0		
(Roman Meal):				
Regular	1-oz. slice	.7	.1	
Light	.8-oz. slice	.2		
White, enriched or unenriched:				
America's Own cottage	1 oz.	1.0		
(Arnold):				
Brick Oven	1 slice (.8 oz.)	1.0		
Country	1.3-oz. slice	0.0		
Very thin	.5-oz. slice	1.0		
Eddy's	1-oz. slice	1.0		
(Monk's)	1-oz.	1.0		
(Pepperidge Farm):				
Regular	1.2-oz. slice	1.5		
Very thin slice	.6-oz. slice	.5		
Whole wheat:				
(Monks') stone ground	1 oz.	1.0		
(Pepperidge Farm) fresh or				
frozen, thin sliced	.9-oz. slice	1.5		
(Roman Meal) 100%	1-oz. slice	.9	.1	
BREAD, CANNED (B&M)				
plain or raisin	½" slice	Tr.		
BREAD CRUMBS:				
(USDA) Dry, grated	1 cup (3.5 oz.)	4.6	1.0	4.0
(USDA) Dry, grated	1 T. (6 grams)	.3	Tr.	Tr.
(Contadina):				
Seasoned	1 rnd. T.	.3		
Seasoned	½ cup (2.1 oz.)	1.8		
(4-C) plain or seasoned	1 T.	Tr.		
(Progresso) any style	1 T.	Tr.		
BREAD DOUGH:				
Frozen:				
(Pepperidge Farm):				
Rye, country	1/10 of loaf	2.0		
Wheat, stone ground or				
white	1/10 of loaf	1.5		
(Rich's):				
French	1/20 of loaf	.6		
Italian or raisin	1/20 of loaf	1.0		
White	.8-oz. serving	.6		
Refrigerated (Pillsbury):				
French	1" slice	<1.0	Tr.	0.0
Wheat or white	1" slice	2.0	<1.0	0.0
BREADFRUIT, fresh (USDA)				
peeled & trimmed	4 oz.	.3		
*BREAD MIX:				
Home Hearth:				
French	3/8" slice	1.5		
Rye or white	3/8" slice	.5		
(Pillsbury):				
Banana or nut	1/12 of loaf	6.0		
Blueberry nut or cranberry	1/12 of loaf	4.0		
BREAD STICK:				
(USDA):				
Salt or Vienna type	1 piece (3 grams)	< .1	Tr.	Tr.
(Stella D'Oro) regular or die-				
tetic:				
Plain, onion, pizza or wheat	1 piece	1.0		
Sesame	1 piece	2.0		

FOOD DESCRIPTION	MEASURE OR QUANTITY	FATS IN GRAMS		
		Total	Saturated	Unsaturated
*BREAD STICK DOUGH, refrigerated:				
(Pillsbury) soft	1 piece	2.0	<1.0	0.0
(Roman Meal)	1.4-oz. piece	3.9	1.2	
BRIGHT & EARLY	6 fl. oz.	.2		
BRITOS, frozen (Patio):				
Beef & bean, chicken, chili, or nacho cheese	½ of 7¼-oz. pkg.	10.0		
Nacho beef	½ of 7¼-oz. pkg.	13.0		
BROADBEAN:				
Immature seed (USDA)	1 oz. (without pod)	.1		
Mature seed, dry (USDA)	1 oz.	.5		
Canned, regular pack, drained solids (Del Monte)	½ cup (2.5 oz.)	< .1		
Frozen (Birds Eye)	⅓ of 9-oz. pkg.	.1		
BROCCOLI:				
Raw, large leaves removed (USDA)	1 lb. (weighed partially trimmed)	1.1		
Boiled without salt, drained (USDA):				
Whole stalk	1 stalk (6.3 oz.)	.5		
½" pieces	½ cup (2.8 oz.)	.2		
Frozen: (USDA):				
Chopped or cut, boiled without salt, drained	1⅜ cups (10-oz. pkg.)	.8		
Spears, boiled without salt, drained	½ cup (3.3 oz.)	.2		
(Birds Eye):				
With almonds and selected seasonings	⅓ of 10-oz. pkg.	2.8		
Cuts or deluxe florets	⅓ of 10-oz. pkg.	.2		
Spears, regular	⅓ of 10-oz. pkg.	.2		
(Green Giant): Cut: In cream sauce:				
Regular	⅓ of 10-oz. pkg.	1.7	<1.0	<1.0
One serving	5-oz. pkg.	3.0	<1.0	0.0
Harvest Fresh	⅓ of 9-oz. pkg.	0.0		
Spears: Butter sauce:				
Regular	⅓ of 10-oz. pkg.	2.0	<1.0	0.0
One serving	4½-oz. pkg.	2.0	<1.0	0.0
Harvest Fresh	⅓ of 9-oz. pkg.	0.0		
BRUSSELS SPROUT:				
Boiled without salt, 1¼–1½" dia., drained (USDA)	1 cup (7–8 sprouts, 5.5 oz.)	.6		
Frozen: (Birds Eye):				
Regular	⅓ of 10-oz. pkg.	.3		
With cheese sauce	⅓ of 9-oz. pkg.	6.8		
(Green Giant):				
Butter sauce	½ cup	1.0	<1.0	0.0
Polybag	½ cup	0.0		
BUCKWHEAT:				
Flour (See FLOUR)				
Groats, *Wolffs* (Birkett)	1 oz.	.5		
Whole grain (USDA)	1 oz.	.7		
BULGUR (from hard red winter wheat) (USDA):				
Dry	1 lb.	6.8		
Canned, seasoned	1 cup (4.8 oz.)	4.5		
Canned, unseasoned	4 oz.	.8		
BUN (See ROLL)				
BURBOT, raw (USDA) meat only	4 oz.	1.0		
BURGER KING:				
Apple pie	1 piece	12.0		
Breakfast Croissantwich:				
Bacon	1 serving	24.0		

FOOD DESCRIPTION	MEASURE OR QUANTITY	FATS IN GRAMS		
		Total	Saturated	Unsaturated
Ham	1 serving	20.0		
Sausage	1 serving	41.0		
Cheeseburger:				
Regular	1 cheeseburger	15.0		
Double:				
Plain	1 burger	27.0		
Bacon	1 burger	31.0		
Chicken Specialty Sandwich, plain	1 sandwich	20.0		
Chicken Tenders	1 piece	1.7		
Coffee, regular	Any quantity	0.0		
Danish, great	1 piece	36.0		
Egg platter, scrambled:				
Bacon	1 serving	6.0		
Croissant or hash browns	1 serving	11.0		
Sausage	1 serving	22.0		
French fries	1 reg. order	13.0		
French toast sticks	1 serving	29.0		
Ham & cheese, specialty sandwich, plain	1 sandwich	13.0		
Hamburger, plain	1 burger	12.0		
Milk:				
2% low-fat	1 serving	5.0		
Whole	1 serving	9.0		
Onion rings	1 serving	16.0		
Orange juice	Any quantity	0.0		
Salad dressing:				
Regular:				
Bleu cheese	1 serving	16.0		
House	1 serving	13.0		
Thousand island	1 serving	12.0		
Dietetic, Italian	1 serving	0.0		
Shake:				
Chocolate	1 shake	12.0		
Strawberry or vanilla	1 shake	10.0		
Soft drink, sweetened or dietetic	Any quantity	0.0		
Whaler, fish sandwich, plain	1 sandwich	13.0		
Whopper:				
Regular:				
Plain	1 burger	21.0		
With cheese	1 burger	28.0		
Junior:				
Plain	1 burger	12.0		
With cheese	1 burger	15.0		
BURGUNDY WINE	Any quantity	0.0		
BURRITO:				
*Canned (Old El Paso)	1 burrito	13.0	4.0	2.0
Frozen:				
Little Juan (Fred's Frozen Foods):				
Bean & cheese	5-oz. serving	9.7		
Beef & bean, spicy	10-oz. serving	39.2		
Chili:				
Green	10-oz. serving	32.7		
Red	10-oz. serving	35.2		
Chili dog	5-oz. serving	14.1		
Red hot	5-oz. serving	21.1		
(Old El Paso):				
Regular:				
Bean & cheese	1 piece	13.0		
Beef & bean, hot or medium	1 piece	14.0		
Dinner, beef & bean, festive	11-oz. dinner	9.0		
(Patio):				
Beef & bean:				
Regular	5-oz. serving	16.0		
Red chili	5-oz. serving	13.0		
Red hot	5-oz. serving	15.0		

FOOD DESCRIPTION	MEASURE OR QUANTITY	FATS IN GRAMS		
		Total	Saturated	Unsaturated
(Van de Kamp's):				
Regular, crispy fried	6-oz. serving	15.0		
Grande, with rice & corn	16¾-oz. pkg.	20.0		
(Weight Watchers):				
Beefsteak	7.6-oz. serving	12.0	4.0	8.0
Chicken	7.6-oz. serving	13.0	4.0	9.0
BURRITO SEASONING mix				
(Lawry's)	1½-oz. pkg.	1.7		
BUTTER:				
Regular:				
(USDA)	¼ lb. (1 stick, ½ cup)	92.0	52.0	40.0
(USDA)	1 T. (⅛ stick, .5 oz.)	11.3	6.0	5.0
(USDA)	1 pat (1″ × 1″ × ⅓″, 5 grams)	4.0	2.0	2.0
(Land O'Lakes)	1 T.	12.0	6.0	<6.0
Whipped:				
(USDA)	2.7 oz. (1 stick, ½ cup)	61.6	35.0	27.0
(USDA)	1 T. (⅛ stick, 9 grams)	7.3	4.0	3.0
(Breakstone's)	1 T. (9 grams)	7.4		
(Land O'Lakes)	1 T.	9.0	6.0	<6.0
BUTTER BEAN (See **BEAN, LIMA**)				
BUTTERFISH, raw (USDA):				
Gulf, meat only	4 oz.	3.3		
Northern, meat only	4 oz.	11.6		
BUTTERMILK (See **MILK**)				
BUTTERNUT (USDA) shelled	4 oz.	11.6		
BUTTER OIL or dehydrated butter (USDA)	1 cup (7.2 oz.)	203.0	112.0	91.0
BUTTERSCOTCH MORSELS (Nestlé) artificial	1 oz.	15.0	7.0	
BUTTER SUBSTITUTE, *Butter-Buds*	Any quantity	0.0		
CABBAGE:				
White or savoy (USDA):				
Raw:				
Whole	1 lb. (weighed untrimmed)	.7		
Coarsely shredded or sliced	1 cup (2.5 oz.)	.1		
Wedge	3½″ × 4½″ wedge (3.5 oz.)	.2		
Boiled until tender:				
Shredded, small amount of water, drained	½ cup (2.6 oz.)	.1		
Wedges, in large amount of water, drained	½ cup (3.2 oz.)	.2		
Red, canned (Comstock-Greenwood)	4 oz.	Tr.		
CABBAGE, CHINESE OR CELERY, raw (USDA) 1″ pieces, leaves with stalk	½ cup (1.3 oz.)	Tr.		
CABBAGE, SPOON OR WHITE MUSTARD OR PAKCHOY (USDA):				
Raw	1 lb. (weighed untrimmed)	.9		
Boiled without salt, drained	½ cup (1.3 oz.)	.2		
CABBAGE STUFFED, frozen (Stouffer's) *Lean Cuisine,* with meat, in tomato sauce	10¾-oz. pkg.	10.0		
CAKE (Some cakes are listed by brand name such as *Bear Claws,* etc.):				
Home Recipe (USDA):				
Plain:				
Without icing:				
Made with butter	⅑ of 9″ sq. cake (3″ × 3″ × 1″-3 oz.)	10.9	6.0	6.0
Made with vegetable shortening	⅑ of 9″ sq. cake (3″ × 3″ × 1″-3 oz.)	12.0	3.0	8.0

FOOD DESCRIPTION	MEASURE OR QUANTITY	FATS IN GRAMS		
		Total	Saturated	Unsaturated
With boiled white icing:				
Made with butter	1/9 of 9" sq. cake (4 oz.)	12.0	7.0	5.0
Made with vegetable shortening	1/9 of 9" sq. cake (4 oz.)	12.0	3.0	9.0
With chocolate icing:				
Made with butter	1/16 of 10" layer cake (3.5 oz.)	12.7	8.0	6.0
Made with vegetable shortening	1/16 of 10" layer cake (3.5 oz.)	12.9	4.0	9.0
Angel food	1/12 of 8" cake	< .1		
Caramel:				
Without icing	1/9 of 9" sq. cake	14.9	8.0	7.0
With caramel icing	3 oz.	12.6		
Chocolate:				
Without icing:				
Made with butter	3 oz.	14.6	8.0	7.0
Made with vegetable shortening	3 oz.	14.6	4.0	10.0
With chocolate icing, 2-layer	1/16 of 10" cake (4.2 oz.)	19.7		
With chocolate icing, 2-layer	1/16 of 9" cake (2.6 oz.)	12.3		
With uncooked white icing	1/16 of 10" cake (4.2 oz.)	17.5		
Devil's food:				
Without icing	3" × 2" × 1 1/2" piece (1.9 oz.)	9.5		
With chocolate icing, 2-layer	1/16 of 9" cake (2.6 oz.)	12.3		
Fruit cake:				
Dark, home recipe	1-lb. loaf	69.4		
Light, home recipe, made with butter	1-lb. loaf	71.2	26.0	45.0
Light, home recipe, made with vegetable shortening	1-lb. loaf	74.8	16.0	59.0
Pound cake:				
Home recipe, old-fashioned, equal weights flour, sugar, eggs & butter	1.1-oz. slice (3 1/2" × 3" × 1/2")	7.9	4.0	4.0
Home recipe, old-fashioned, equal weights flour, sugar, eggs & vegetable shortening	1.1-oz. slice (3 1/2" × 3" × 1/2")	8.8	2.0	7.0
Home recipe, traditional, made with vegetable shortening	1.1-oz. slice (3 1/2" × 3" × 1/2")	5.6	2.0	4.0
White:				
Without icing:				
Made with butter	1/9 of 9" sq. cake (3" × 3" × 1"-3 oz.)	13.8	8.0	6.0
Made with vegetable shortening	1/9 of 9" sq. cake (3" × 3" × 1"-3 oz.)	13.8	4.0	10.0
With uncooked white icing:				
Made with butter	1/16 of 10" layer cake (3.5 oz.)	12.9	7.0	6.0
Made with vegetable shortening	1/16 of 10" layer cake (3.5 oz.)	12.9	5.0	9.0
Yellow:				
Without icing:				
Made with butter	1/9 of 9" sq. cake (3" × 3" × 1" – 3 oz.)	10.9	6.0	5.0

FOOD DESCRIPTION	MEASURE OR QUANTITY	FATS IN GRAMS		
		Total	**Saturated**	**Unsaturated**
Made with vegetable shortening	1/9 of 9″ sq. cake (3″ × 3″ × 1″-3 oz.)	10.9	3.0	8.0
With caramel icing:				
Made with butter	1/16 of 10″ layer cake (3.5 oz.)	11.7	6.0	6.0
Made with vegetable shortening	1/16 of 10″ layer cake (3.5 oz.)	11.7	3.0	9.0
With chocolate icing, 2-layer:				
Made with butter	1/16 of 9″ cake	9.8	6.0	4.0
Made with vegetable shortening	1/16 of 9″ cake (2.6 oz.)	9.8	3.0	7.0
Commercial type:				
Not frozen:				
Angel food (Dolly Madison) bar	1/6 of 10.5-oz. cake	5.0		
Apple:				
(Dolly Madison) dutch, *Buttercrumb*	1½-oz. piece	6.0		
(Entenmann's) spice-, fat- & cholesterol-free	1-oz. slice	0.0		
Banana crunch (Entenmann's) fat- & cholesterol-free	1-oz. slice	0.0		
Blueberry crunch (Entenmann's) fat- & cholesterol-free	1-oz. slice	0.0		
Butter streusel (Dolly Madison) *Buttercrumb*	1½-oz. piece	6.0		
Carrot (Dolly Madison) *Lunch Cake*	3¼-oz. serving	9.0		
Chocolate:				
(Dolly Madison) German, *Lunch Cake*	3¼-oz. serving	17.0		
(Entenmann's) loaf, fat- & cholesterol-free	1-oz. slice	0.0		
Cinnamon (Dolly Madison) *Buttercrumb*	1½-oz. piece	8.0		
Coffee (Entenmann's) fat- & cholesterol-free, cherry or cinnamon apple	1.3-oz. piece	0.0		
Creme (Dolly Madison) *Lunch Cake*	7/8-oz. piece	3.0		
Golden (Entenmann's) loaf, fat- & cholesterol-free	1-oz. slice	0.0		
Hawaiian spice (Dolly Madison) *Lunch Cake*	3¼-oz. serving	12.0		
Honey'n Spice (Dolly Madison) *Lunch Cake*	3¼-oz. serving	10.0		
Pineapple crunch (Entenmann's) fat- & cholesterol-free	1-oz. slice	0.0		
Pound (Dolly Madison)	1/6 of 14-oz. cake	8.0		
White (Dolly Madison) coconut layer	1/12 of 30-oz. cake	7.0		
Frozen:				
Black forest (Weight Watchers)	3-oz. serving	5.0	1.0	4.0
Boston cream:				
(Pepperidge Farm)	1/4 of 11¾-oz. cake	14.0		
(Weight Watchers)	3-oz. serving	4.0	1.0	3.0
Carrot:				
(Pepperidge Farm) with cream-cheese icing	1/8 of 11¾-oz. cake	8.0		
(Weight Watchers)	3-oz. serving	5.0	<1.0	5.0

FOOD DESCRIPTION	MEASURE OR QUANTITY	FATS IN GRAMS		
		Total	Saturated	Unsaturated
Cheese (Weight Watchers):				
Regular	3-oz. serving	7.0	1.0	6.0
Strawberry	3.9-oz. serving	5.0	1.0	4.0
Chocolate:				
(Pepperidge Farm) layer, fudge	1/10 of 17-oz. cake	10.0		
(Weight Watchers):				
Regular	2½-oz. serving	5.0	<1.0	5.0
German	2½-oz. serving	7.0	<1.0	7.0
Coconut (Pepperidge Farm)	1/10 of 17-oz. cake	9.0		
Devil's food (Pepperidge Farm)	1/10 of 17-oz. cake	9.0		
Lemon coconut (Pepperidge Farm) supreme	1/4 of 12¼-oz. cake	13.0		
Pound (Pepperidge Farm)	1/10 of 10¾-oz. cake	7.0		
Vanilla (Pepperidge Farm)	1/10 of 17-oz. cake	8.0		
CAKE ICING:				
Butter pecan (Betty Crocker) *Creamy Deluxe*	1/12 of pkg.	7.0	2.0	<5.0
Caramel pecan (Pillsbury) *Frosting Supreme*	1/12 of pkg.	8.0		
Cherry (Betty Crocker) *Creamy Deluxe*	1/12 of pkg.	6.0	2.0	<4.0
Chocolate:				
(Betty Crocker) *Creamy Deluxe:*				
Regular	1/12 of pkg.	7.0	2.0	<5.0
Chip or sour cream	1/12 of pkg.	7.0	3.0	<5.0
Fudge, dark dutch	1/12 of pkg.	6.0	2.0	<4.0
(Duncan Hines) regular, dark dutch fudge or milk	1/12 of pkg.	6.3		
(Pillsbury) *Frosting Supreme,* chip	1/12 of pkg.	5.0		
Coconut, home recipe (USDA)	1 cup (5.8 oz.)	12.8	12.0	Tr.
Coconut pecan (Pillsbury) *Frosting Supreme*	1/12 of pkg.	10.0		
Cream cheese:				
(Betty Crocker) *Creamy Deluxe*	1/12 of pkg.	6.0	2.0	<4.0
(Duncan Hines)	1/12 of pkg.	6.3		
Double Dutch (Pillsbury) *Frosting Supreme*	1/12 of pkg.	6.0		
Lemon (Betty Crocker) *Creamy Deluxe*	1/12 of pkg.	6.0	2.0	<4.0
Polka dot (Duncan Hines) milk chocolate	1/12 of pkg.	7.4		
Rocky Road (Betty Crocker) *Creamy Deluxe*	1/12 of pkg.	8.0	2.0	6.0
Strawberry (Pillsbury) *Frosting Supreme*	1/12 of pkg.	6.0		
Vanilla:				
(Betty Crocker) *Creamy Deluxe*	1/12 of pkg.	6.0	2.0	<4.0
(Pillsbury) *Frosting Supreme,* regular or sour cream	1/12 of pkg.	6.0		
White:				
Home recipe (USDA):				
Boiled	1 cup (3.3 oz.)	0.0		
Uncooked	4 oz.	7.5	4.0	3.0
(Betty Crocker) *Creamy Deluxe,* sour cream	1/12 of pkg.	6.0	2.0	<4.0
*CAKE ICING MIX:				
Chocolate:				
(Betty Crocker) creamy:				
Fudge	1/12 of pkg.	6.0	2.0	4.0

FOOD DESCRIPTION	MEASURE OR QUANTITY	FATS IN GRAMS		
		Total	Saturated	Unsaturated
Milk	1/12 of pkg.	5.0	1.0	4.0
(Pillsbury) *Frost It Hot*	1/8 of pkg.	0.0		
Coconut pecan (Betty Crocker) creamy	1/12 of pkg.	8.0	3.0	5.0
Lemon (Betty Crocker) creamy	1/12 of pkg.	6.0		
Vanilla:				
(Betty Crocker)	1/12 of pkg.	5.0	1.0	4.0
(Pillsbury) *Frosting Supreme*, regular or sour cream	1/12 of pkg.	6.0		
White:				
(Betty Crocker):				
Regular, creamy	1/12 of pkg.	6.0		
Fluffy	1/12 of pkg.	0.0		
(Pillsbury) fluffy:				
Regular	1/12 of pkg.	0.0		
Frost It Hot	1/8 of pkg.	0.0		
CAKE MIX:				
Regular:				
Angel food:				
(Betty Crocker) any type	1/12 of pkg.	0.0		
(Duncan Hines)	1/12 of pkg.	.1		
*Apple cinnamon (Betty Crocker) *Supermoist:*				
Regular recipe	1/12 of cake	10.0		
No-cholesterol recipe	1/12 of cake	6.0		
*Banana (Pillsbury) *Pillsbury Plus*	1/12 of cake	11.0		
*Boston cream (Pillsbury) *Bundt*	1/16 of cake	10.0		
*Butter (Pillsbury) *Pillsbury Plus*	1/12 of cake	12.0		
*Butter pecan (Betty Crocker) *Supermoist:*				
Regular recipe	1/12 of cake	11.0		
No-cholesterol recipe	1/12 of cake	7.0		
*Carrot (Betty Crocker) *Supermoist:*				
Regular recipe	1/12 of cake	11.0		
No-cholesterol recipe	1/12 of cake	7.0		
*Cheesecake:				
(Jell-O)	1/8 of cake	12.0		
(Royal) No Bake:				
Lite	1/8 of cake	10.0		
Real	1/8 of cake	9.0		
Chocolate:				
*(Betty Crocker):				
MicroRave:				
Fudge, with vanilla frosting	1/6 of cake	15.0	4.0	11.0
German, with coconut pecan frosting	1/6 of cake	18.0	5.0	13.0
Pudding recipe	1/6 of cake	6.0		
Supermoist:				
Chip:				
Regular recipe	1/12 of cake	14.0	3.0	11.0
No-cholesterol recipe	1/12 of cake	7.0	2.0	5.0
Fudge	1/12 of cake	12.0	3.0	9.0
Milk:				
Regular recipe	1/12 of cake	12.0	3.0	9.0
No-cholesterol recipe	1/12 of cake	7.0	2.0	5.0
(Duncan Hines) fudge, butter recipe	1/12 of pkg.	4.2		
*(Pillsbury):				
Bundt:				
Fudge, tunnel of	1/16 of cake	12.0		
Macaroon	1/16 of cake	10.0		

FOOD DESCRIPTION	MEASURE OR QUANTITY	FATS IN GRAMS		
		Total	Saturated	Unsaturated
Microwave:				
Regular:				
Plain	⅛ of cake	13.0		
With chocolate or vanilla frosting	⅛ of cake	17.0		
Double, supreme	⅛ of cake	19.0		
Pillsbury Plus:				
Chip	1/12 of cake	14.0		
Dark or marble fudge	1/12 of cake	12.0		
*Coffee cake:				
(Aunt Jemima)	⅛ of cake	.6		
(Pillsbury) apple cinnamon	⅛ of cake	7.0		
Devil's Food:				
*(Betty Crocker):				
MicroRave, with chocolate frosting:				
Regular recipe	⅙ of cake	17.0	5.0	12.0
No-cholesterol recipe	⅙ of cake	9.0	3.0	6.0
Supermoist:				
Regular recipe	1/12 of cake	12.0	3.0	9.0
No-cholesterol recipe	1/12 of cake	7.0	2.0	5.0
*(Pillsbury) *Pillsbury Plus*	1/12 of cake	14.0		
Fudge (See Chocolate)				
Lemon:				
*(Betty Crocker):				
MicroRave, with lemon frosting	⅙ of cake	16.0	4.0	12.0
Supermoist no-cholesterol recipe	1/12 of cake	7.0	2.0	5.0
*(Pillsbury):				
Microwave:				
Regular	⅛ of cake	13.0		
With lemon frosting	⅛ of cake	17.0		
Pillsbury Plus	1/12 of cake	11.0		
*Marble (Betty Crocker) *Supermoist:*				
Regular recipe	1/12 of cake	11.0	3.0	8.0
No-cholesterol recipe	1/12 of cake	7.0	2.0	5.0
*Pound:				
(Betty Crocker) golden	1/12 of cake	9.0	3.0	6.0
(Dromedary)	½" slice	6.0		
*Upside down cake (Betty Crocker) pineapple	⅑ of cake	10.0	4.0	< 6.0
*Vanilla (Betty Crocker):				
MicroRave, golden, with rainbow chip frosting	⅙ of cake	17.0	5.0	12.0
Supermoist, golden:				
Regular recipe	1/12 of cake	14.0	3.0	11.0
No-cholesterol recipe	1/12 of cake	7.0	2.0	5.0
White:				
*(Betty Crocker) *Supermoist:*				
Regular	1/12 of cake	9.0	2.0	7.0
Sour cream	1/12 of cake	3.0	1.0	2.0
(Duncan Hines) deluxe	1/12 of pkg.	4.0		
*(Pillsbury) *Pillsbury Plus*	1/12 of cake	10.0		
Yellow:				
*(Betty Crocker):				
MicroRave, with chocolate frosting:				
Regular recipe	⅙ of cake	16.0	4.0	12.0
No-cholesterol recipe	⅙ of cake	9.0	3.0	6.0
Supermoist:				
Regular recipe	1/12 of cake	11.0	3.0	8.0
No-cholesterol recipe	1/12 of cake	7.0	2.0	5.0

FOOD DESCRIPTION	MEASURE OR QUANTITY	FATS IN GRAMS		
		Total	Saturated	Unsaturated
(Duncan Hines) deluxe	1/12 of pkg.	3.6		
*(Pillsbury):				
Microwave:				
Regular	1/8 of cake	13.0		
With chocolate frosting	1/8 of cake	17.0		
Pillsbury Plus	1/12 of cake	12.0		
*Dietetic (Estee)	1/10 of cake	2.0	<1.0	
CANADIAN WHISKEY (See **DISTILLED LIQUOR**)				
CANDY. The following values of candies from the U.S. Department of Agriculture are representative of the types sold commercially. These values may be useful when individual brands or sizes are not known:				
Almond:				
Chocolate-coated	1 oz.	12.4	2.0	10.0
Sugarcoated or Jordan	1 oz.	5.3	Tr.	5.0
Candy corn	1 oz.	.6		
Caramel:				
Plain	1 oz.	2.9	1.0	2.0
Plain with nuts	1 oz.	4.6	2.0	3.0
Chocolate	1 oz.	2.9	1.0	2.0
Chocolate with nuts	1 oz.	4.6	2.0	3.0
Chocolate:				
Bittersweet	1 oz.	11.3	6.0	5.0
Milk:				
Plain	1 oz.	9.2	5.0	4.0
With almonds	1 oz.	10.1		
Semisweet or sweet	1 oz.	10.1	6.0	4.0
Fondant, plain	1 oz.	.6	Tr.	Tr.
Fondant, chocolate-covered	1 oz.	3.0	1.0	2.0
Fudge:				
Chocolate:				
Regular	1 oz.	3.5	1.0	2.0
With nuts	1 oz.	4.9	2.0	3.0
Vanilla:				
Regular	1 oz.	3.1	1.0	2.0
With nuts	1 oz.	4.6	2.0	3.0
Gum drops	1 oz.	.2		
Hard	1 oz.	.3		
Jelly beans	1 oz.	.1		
Marshmallows	1 oz.	Tr.		
Peanut bar	1 oz.	9.1	2.0	7.0
Peanut brittle, no added salt or soda	1 oz.	2.9	<1.0	2.0
Peanuts, chocolate coated	1 oz.	11.7	3.0	9.0
Raisins, chocolate coated	1 oz.	4.8	3.0	2.0
CANDY, COMMERCIAL (See also **CANDY, DIETETIC**):				
Almond Joy (Hershey's)	1.76-oz. bar	14.0		
Baby Ruth (Nabisco)	2-oz. serving	12.0		
Bar-None (Hershey's)	1.5-oz. serving	14.0		
Bit-O-Honey (Nestlé)	1-oz. serving	2.0		
Bridge Mix (Nabisco)	1 piece (2 grams)	.4		
Butterfinger (Nab)	2-oz. serving	12.0		
Caramel Nip (Pearson)	1 piece (.25 oz.)	.7		
Caramello (Hershey's)	1.6-oz. bar	11.0		
Charleston Chew!	2-oz. serving	6.0		
Cherry, chocolate-covered (Welch's) Cortina, dark or milk	3/4-oz. piece	2.0		
Chocolate bar:				
Alpine white (Nestlé)	1-oz. serving	12.0		
Brazil nut, Cadbury's (Peter Paul)	2-oz. serving	18.0		
Crunch (Nestlé)	1 1/16-oz. bar	8.0		

FOOD DESCRIPTION	MEASURE OR QUANTITY	FATS IN GRAMS		
		Total	Saturated	Unsaturated
Milk:				
(Hershey's)	1.55-oz. bar	14.0		
(Nestlé)	1 1/15-oz. bar	8.5		
Special Dark (Hershey's)	1.45-oz. bar	12.0		
Chocolate bar with almonds:				
Cadbury's (Peter Paul)	2-oz. bar	18.0		
(Hershey's) milk	1.45-oz. bar	14.0		
(Nestlé)	1-oz. serving	8.0		
Chocolate Parfait (Pearson)	.25-oz. piece	.7		
Chuckles, any flavor	1 oz.	0.0		
Chunky (Nestlé):				
Regular	1 oz.	8.0		
Deluxe nut	1 oz.	10.0		
Coffee Nip (Pearson)	.25-oz. piece	.7		
Creme De Menthe's (Andes)	.2-oz. piece	1.5	1.4	.15
Eggs (Peter Paul)	1 oz.	6.0		
Fifth Avenue (Hershey's)	2.1-oz. serving	13.0		
Fruit Bears (Flavor Tree) as-sorted	1/2 of 2.1-oz. pkg.	1.6		
Fruit Circus (Flavor Tree) as-sorted	1/2 of 2.1-oz. pkg.	1.6		
Goobers (Nestlé)	1 oz.	10.0		
Halvah (Sahadi)	1 oz.	10.0		
Hard (Jolly Rancher)	1 piece	Tr.		
Holidays (M&M/Mars):				
Plain	1 oz.	6.0		
Peanut	1 oz.	7.0		
Jelly, *Chuckles:*				
Bar or bean	1 oz.	0.0		
Rings	1 oz.	1.0		
Jujubes (Nabisco) *Chuckles*	1/2 oz.	Tr.		
Kisses (Hershey's) plain	1 piece (5 grams)	1.4		
Kit Kat (Hershey's)	1.6-oz. bar	13.0		
Krackel (Hershey's)	1.55-oz. bar	13.0		
Licorice:				
Licorice Nip (Pearson)	.25-oz. piece	.7		
(Switzer's) bars, bites or stix	1 oz.	Tr.		
Life Savers	1 piece	0.0		
Lollipop, *Life Savers*	1 piece	0.0		
Mars (M&M/Mars)	1.76-oz. bar	11.0		
Mary Jane (Miller):				
Small	7.3-gram piece	< .1	Tr.	Tr.
Large	1 1/4-oz. piece	.4	Tr.	Tr.
Milky Way (M&M/Mars) milk chocolate	2.24-oz. bar	11.0		
Mint or peppermint:				
Canada Mint (Necco)	.1-oz. piece	Tr.		
Mint parfait (Andes)	.2-oz. piece	1.6	1.2	.4
Pattie:				
(Nabisco):				
Regular	1 piece	Tr.		
Chocolate-covered, Junior	2.4-gram piece	.2		
York (Hersey's) choco-late-covered	1.5-oz. piece	4.0		
M&M's (M&M/Mars):				
Plain	1.7-oz. pkg.	10.0		
Peanut	1.8-oz. pkg.	13.0		
Mounds (Hershey's)	1.9-oz. piece	14.0		
Mr. Goodbar (Hershey's)	1.85-oz. bar	19.0		
Necco Wafers	2.02-oz. roll	0.0		
Oh Henry! (Nestlé)	1 oz.	4.0		
$100,000 (Nestlé)	1.5-oz. bar	8.0		
Orange slice, *Chuckles* (Nabisco)	1 oz.	1.0		
Park Avenue (Tom's)	1.8-oz. serving	9.0		
Peanut butter cup (Reese's)	9-oz. piece	8.0		
Peanut Butter Pals (Tom's)	1.3-oz. piece	11.0		

FOOD DESCRIPTION	MEASURE OR QUANTITY	FATS IN GRAMS		
		Total	Saturated	Unsaturated
Peanut parfait:				
(Andes)	5-gram piece	1.8	1.1	.7
(Pearson's)	.25-oz. piece	.7		
Peanut Plank (Tom's)	1.7-oz. serving	11.0		
Power House (Peter Paul)	2-oz. serving	11.0		
Raisin, chocolate-covered				
(Nabisco)	1 piece	.2		
Raisinets (Nestlé)	1 oz.	4.0		
Reese's Pieces (Hershey's)	1.95-oz. pkg.	11.0		
Rolo (Hershey's)	.2-oz. piece	1.5		
Royals (M&M/Mars)	1.52-oz. pkg.	9.0		
Sesame crunch bar (Sahadi)	¾-oz. bar	7.0		
Skittles (M&M/Mars)	1 oz.	.9		
Sky bar (Necco)	1.5-oz. bar	7.2		
Snickers (M&M/Mars)	2.16-oz. bar	14.0		
Solitaires (Hershey's)	3.2-oz. pkg.	17.0		
Spearmint leaves, Chuckles				
(Nabisco)	1 oz.	1.0		
Starburst (M&M/Mars)	1 oz.	2.5		
Stars, chocolate (Nabisco)	2.2-gram piece	.6		
Sugar Babies (Nabisco)	1⅝-oz. serving	2.0		
Sugar Daddy (Nabisco)	1⅜-oz. piece	1.0		
Symphony (Hershey's):				
Almond	1.4-oz. piece	14.0		
Milk	1.4-oz. piece	13.0		
3 Musketeers bar (M&M/ Mars)	2.13-oz. bar	8.0		
Tootsie Roll:				
Regular:				
Chocolate	1 oz.	2.5		
Flavored	.23-oz. piece	.5		
Pop:				
Caramel	.49-oz. piece	.5		
Chocolate or flavored	.49-oz. piece	.3		
Pop drop	.2-oz. piece	.2		
Whatchamacallit (Hershey's)	1.8-oz. bar	13.0		
Y&S Bites (Hershey's)	1 oz.	1.0		
CANDY, DIETETIC:				
Caramel (Estee)	1 piece	1.0	< 1.0	
Carob bar, Joan's Natural:				
Coconut	3-oz. piece	41.8		
Honey bran	3-oz. piece	35.1		
Chocolate bar (Estee):				
Coconut	.2-oz. square	2.5		
Crunch	.2-oz. square	1.5		
Fruit & nut, or milk	.2-oz. square	2.0	1.5	
Estee-ets (Estee) with peanuts	1 piece	.4		
Gum drop (Estee) fruit or licorice	1 piece	Tr.		
Gummy Bears (Estee)	1 piece	0.0		
Hard (Estee) assorted	1 piece	Tr.		
Peanut brittle (Estee)	¼ oz.	1.0		
Peanut butter cup (Estee)	7.7-gram piece	3.0	2.5	
CANE SYRUP (See **SYRUP,** Cane)				
CANNELLONI, frozen:				
(Celetano) florentine	12-oz. pkg.	8.0		
(Stouffer's) Lean Cuisine:				
Beef & pork, with mornay sauce	9⅝-oz. pkg.	10.0		
Cheese with tomato sauce	9⅛-oz. pkg.	10.0		
CANTALOUPE, fresh:				
Whole, medium (USDA)	5" dia. melon (1⅔ lbs., weighed with skin & cavity contents)	.4		
Cubed (USDA)	½ cup (2.9 oz.)	< .1		
CAPICOLA OR CAPACOLA SAUSAGE (USDA)	1 oz.	13.0	5.0	8.0

FOOD DESCRIPTION	MEASURE OR QUANTITY	FATS IN GRAMS		
		Total	Saturated	Unsaturated
CAP'N CRUNCH, cereal (Quaker):				
Regular or *Crunch Berries*	¾ cup (1 oz.)	2.6		
Peanut butter	¾ cup (1 oz.)	3.8		
CARL'S JR. RESTAURANT :				
Bacon	2 strips (10 grams)	4.0	3.0	Tr.
Cake, chocolate	3.2-oz. piece	20.0		
California Roast Beef'n Swiss Sandwich	7.2-oz. sandwich	8.0		
Cheese:				
American	.6-oz. slice	5.0		
Swiss	.6-oz. slice	4.0		
Cheeseburger, Western Bacon:				
Regular	7½-oz. serving	33.0		
Double	10.4-oz. serving	53.0		
Chicken sandwich:				
Charbroiler BBQ	6.3-oz. sandwich	5.0	5.0	
Charbroiler Club	8.2-oz. sandwich	85.0		
Cookie, chocolate chip	2¼-oz. piece	13.0		
Hot cakes, with margarine, excluding syrup	5.5-oz. serving	12.0		
Muffins:				
Blueberry	3.5-oz. piece	7.0		
Bran	4-oz. piece	6.0		
English, with margarine	2-oz. piece	6.0		
Onion rings	1 regular order	15.0		
Potato:				
Baked:				
Bacon & cheese	14.1-oz. serving	34.0		
Broccoli & cheese	14-oz. serving	17.0		
Cheese	14.2-oz. serving	22.0		
Lite	9.8-oz. serving	3.0		
Sour cream & chive	10.4-oz. serving	13.0		
French fries	regular order (6 oz.)	17.0		
Hash brown nuggets	3-oz. serving	9.0		
Salad dressing:				
Regular:				
Blue cheese	2-oz. serving	14.0		
House	2-oz. serving	17.0		
Thousand island	2-oz. serving	23.0		
Dietetic, Italian	2-oz. serving	10.0		
Sausage patty	1.5-oz. piece	17.0		
Shake	1 regular size	7.0		
Soft drink, sweetened or dietetic	1 regular size	0.0		
Soup:				
Chicken & noodle	1 serving	1.0		
Clam chowder, Boston	1 serving	8.0		
Vegetable, mixed	1 serving	2.0		
Steak sandwich, Country Fried	7.2-oz. serving	33.0		
Sunrise Sandwich:				
Bacon	4.5-oz. serving	19.0		
Sausage	6.1-oz. serving	32.0		
Zucchini	4.3-oz. serving	16.0		
CARNATION DO-IT-YOURSELF DIET PLAN:				
Chocolate	1 scoop (1.1 oz.)	1.0		
Vanilla	2 scoops (1.1 oz.)	.5		
CARNATION INSTANT BREAKFAST:				
Bar:				
Chocolate chip, honey nut, peanut butter with chocolate chips or peanut butter crunch	1 bar	11.0		
Chocolate Crunch	1 bar	10.0		

FOOD DESCRIPTION	MEASURE OR QUANTITY	FATS IN GRAMS		
		Total	Saturated	Unsaturated
*Dry:				
Chocolate	8 fl. oz.	10.0		
Chocolate malt	8 fl. oz.	9.0		
CAROB FLOUR (See **FLOUR**)				
CARP, raw (USDA) meat				
only	4 oz.	4.8		
CARROT:				
Raw (USDA):				
Whole	1 lb. (weighed with full tops)	.5		
Partially trimmed	1 lb. (weighed without tops, with skins)	.7		
Trimmed	5½" × 1" carrot (1.8 oz.)	.1		
Chunks, diced, grated or shredded, sliced or strips	½ cup	.1		
Boiled, without salt (USDA):				
Chunks, drained	½ cup (2.9 oz.)	.2		
Diced, drained	½ cup (2.5 oz.)	.1		
Canned, regular pack:				
(USDA) diced, solids & liq.	½ cup (4.3 oz.)	.2		
(Del Monte) diced, sliced or whole, solids & liq.	4 oz.	0.0		
Canned, dietetic pack:				
(Larsen) *Fresh-Lite,* water pack	½ cup (4.4 oz.)	0.0		
(S&W) *Nutradiet,* green label	½ cup	0.0		
Dehydrated (USDA)	1 oz.	.4		
Frozen:				
(Birds Eye) whole, baby, de-luxe	⅓ of 10-oz. pkg.	.2		
(Green Giant) crinkle cut, in butter sauce	½ cup	1.0		
(McKenzie) whole	3.3 oz.	0.0		
With brown-sugar glaze (Birds Eye)	½ cup (3.3 oz.)	2.4		
CASABA MELON, fresh				
(USDA) flesh only	4 oz.	Tr.		
CASHEW NUT:				
(USDA)	1 oz.	13.0	2.0	11.0
(Beer Nuts)	1 oz.	13.0		
(Eagle Snacks):				
Honey Roast:				
Plain	1 oz.	12.0		
With peanuts	1 oz.	13.0		
Lightly salted	1 oz.	14.0		
(Planter's):				
Dry roasted, salted or un-salted	1 oz.	13.0		
Honey roasted, plain or with peanuts	1 oz.	12.0		
Oil roasted, salted or un-salted	1 oz.	14.0		
CASHEW BUTTER (Hain) raw				
or toasted	1 T.	8.0	1.5	2.0
CATAWBA WINE	Any quantity	0.0		
CATFISH:				
Raw (USDA) freshwater, fillet	4 oz.	3.5		
Frozen (Mrs. Paul's) breaded & fried, fillet	3.6-oz. piece	12.0		
CATSUP:				
Regular pack:				
(USDA)	½ cup (5 oz.)	.6		
(USDA)	1 T. (.6 oz.)	Tr.		
(Del Monte)	1 T. (.7 oz.)	Tr.		
(Hunt's)	1 T. (.5 oz.)	Tr.		
Dietetic pack:				
(Hunt's)	1 T. (.5 oz.)	0.0		
(Weight Watchers)	1 T.	0.0		

FOOD DESCRIPTION	MEASURE OR QUANTITY	FATS IN GRAMS		
		Total	Saturated	Unsaturated
CAULIFLOWER:				
Raw (USDA):				
Whole	1 lb. (weighed untrimmed)	.4		
Flowerbuds	1 lb. (weighed trimmed)	.9		
Boiled, without salt, drained (USDA)	½ cup (2.2 oz.)	.1		
Frozen:				
(Birds Eye):				
Regular	⅓ of 10-oz. pkg.	.1		
With cheese sauce	½ of 10-oz. pkg.	7.0		
(Green Giant):				
In cheese sauce:				
Regular	⅓ of 10-oz. pkg.	1.7	Tr.	Tr.
One serving	5½-oz. pkg.	2.0	Tr.	Tr.
Polybag, cuts	½ cup (2 oz.)	0.0		
(Larsen)	3.3 oz.	0.0		
CAVIAR, STURGEON (USDA):				
Pressed	1 oz.	4.7		
Whole eggs	1 oz.	4.3		
CELERY, all varieties:				
Raw (USDA):				
Whole	1 lb. (weighed untrimmed)	.3		
1 large outer stalk	8″ × 1½″ at root end (1.4 oz.)	Tr.		
3 smaller inner stalks	5″ × ¾″ (1.8 oz.)	Tr.		
Diced, chopped, cut in chunks, or sliced	½ cup (1.9 oz.)	Tr.		
Boiled without salt, drained:				
Diced, cut in chunks, or sliced	½ cup (3 oz.)	Tr.		
Frozen (Larsen)	3½ oz.	0.0		
CEREAL BAR (Kellogg's)				
Smart Start:				
Common Sense, oat bran with raspberry filling	1½-oz. bar	6.0		
Corn flakes, with mixed berry filling	1½-oz. bar	7.0		
Nutri-Grain, blueberry or strawberry	1½-oz. bar	8.0		
Rice Krispies, with almonds	1-oz. bar	6.0		
CEREAL BREAKFAST FOODS (See kind of cereal such as **CORN FLAKES** or brand name such as **KIX**)				
CERVELAT (USDA):				
Dry	1 oz.	10.7		
Soft	1 oz.	6.9		
CHABLIS WINE	Any Quantity	0.0		
CHAMPAGNE	Any Quantity	0.0		
CHARLOTTE RUSSE, with ladyfingers, whipped cream filling, home recipe (USDA)	4 oz.	16.6	8.0	9.0
CHEERIOS, cereal (General Mills):				
Regular or apple cinnamon	1 oz.	2.0		
Honey nut	¾ cup (1 oz.)	1.0		
CHEERIOS TO-GO (General Mills):				
Plain or apple cinnamon	1 pouch	2.0		
Honey nut	1 pouch	1.0		
CHEESE:				
American or cheddar:				
Churny Lite, mild or sharp	1 oz.	5.0	3.0	0.0
(Dorman's):				
American:				
Lo-chol	1 oz.	7.0		
Low-sodium	1 oz.	9.0		
Cheddar:				
Light, regular, or *Chedda-Jack*	1 oz.	5.0		
Lo-chol	1 oz.	7.0		

FOOD DESCRIPTION	MEASURE OR QUANTITY	FATS IN GRAMS		
		Total	Saturated	Unsaturated
(Land O'Lakes):				
American, process:				
Regular or sharp	1 oz.	9.0	6.0	<4.0
& swiss	1 oz.	8.0	5.0	<3.0
Cheddar, natural:				
Regular, & bacon or extra-sharp	1 oz.	9.0	6.0	<4.0
Chederella	1 oz.	8.0	5.0	<3.0
(Polly-O) cheddar, shredded	1 oz.	9.0		
Bleu or Blue:				
(USDA) natural:				
Regular	1 oz.	8.6	5.0	4.0
Crumbled	1 cup (4.8 oz.)	41.2	23.0	18.0
(Sargento)	1 oz.	9.1		
Bonbino, Laughing Cow, natural	1 oz.	9.0		
Brick (Land O'Lakes)	1 oz.	8.0	5.0	<3.0
Brie (Sargento) Danish Danko	1 oz.	8.0		
Camembert, domestic (USDA) natural	1 oz.	7.0	4.0	3.0
Cheddar (See American)				
Colby, natural:				
Churny Lite	1 oz.	5.0	3.0	0.0
(Land O'Lakes)	1 oz.	9.0	6.0	<4.0
Cottage:				
Creamed, unflavored:				
(USDA)	1 oz.	1.2	<1.0	<1.0
(USDA)	8-oz. pkg.	9.5	5.0	5.0
(Borden's):				
Regular, 4% milk fat, regular or unsalted	½ cup	5.0		
Lite-Line, 1.5% milk fat	½ cup	2.0		
(Friendship) low-fat, no salt added	1 oz.	.2		
(Johanna Farms):				
Large or small curd	½ cup	4.6		
Low-fat or low-sodium	½ cup	1.0		
(Land O'Lakes)	1 oz.	1.2	.7	< .7
(Weight Watchers) 1% milk fat	½ cup	1.0		
Uncreamed:				
(USDA)	8-oz. pkg.	.7		
(USDA)	1 oz.	< .1		
Cream cheese:				
Plain, unwhipped:				
(USDA)	1 oz.	10.7	6.0	5.0
(USDA)	3-oz. pkg. (2⅞" x ⅞")	32.0	18.0	14.0
(Breakstone's)	1 oz.	9.5		
(Kraft)	1 oz.	9.7		
Plain, whipped (Breakstone's) Temp-Tee	1 oz.	9.5		
Flavored, unwhipped (Kraft):				
Chive, Hostess or Philadelphia Brand	1 oz.	8.0		
Olive-pimento, Hostess	1 oz.	8.3		
Roquefort, Hostess	1 oz.	7.5		
Flavored, whipped (Kraft):				
Bacon & horseradish	1 oz.	9.4		
Chive or onion	1 oz.	8.8		
Pimento	1 oz.	8.6		
Salami or smoked salmon	1 oz.	8.2		
Edam:				
(Land O'Lakes)	1 oz.	8.0	5.0	<3.0
Laughing Cow	1 oz.	8.0		
Farmer:				
(Friendship) regular or no salt added	1 oz.	3.0		
(Sargento)	1 oz.	5.0		

FOOD DESCRIPTION	MEASURE OR QUANTITY	FATS IN GRAMS		
		Total	Saturated	Unsaturated
Feta (Sargento) Danish, cups	1 oz.	6.0		
Gouda:				
(Kaukauna) natural, regular, with caraway seeds or hickory smoked	1 oz.	8.0		
Laughing Cow, natural:				
Regular	1 oz.	9.0		
Mini, waxed	¾ oz.	6.4		
Gruyere (Swiss Knight)	1 oz.	8.0		
Havarti (Sargento) creamy:				
Regular	1 oz.	7.0		
60% milk	1 oz.	10.0		
Hoop (Friendship)		Tr.		
Jalapeño jack (Land O'Lakes)	1 oz.	8.0	5.0	<3.0
Jarlsberg (Sargento) Norwegian	1 oz.	7.0		
Kettle Morain (Sargento)	1 oz.	8.0		
Limburger, natural (USDA)	1 oz.	7.9	4.0	4.0
Monterey Jack:				
Churny Lite	1 oz.	5.0	3.0	0.0
(Land O'Lakes)	1 oz.	9.0	5.0	<4.0
Mozzarella:				
(Dorman's):				
Light	1 oz.	4.0		
Lo-chol	1 oz.	6.0		
(Polly-O):				
Fior de Latte	1 oz.	6.0		
Lite	1 oz.	4.0		
Part skim milk:				
Regular	1 oz.	5.0		
Smoked	1 oz.	7.0		
Whole milk:				
Regular	1 oz.	6.0		
Old-fashioned, regular	1 oz.	4.0		
Muenster:				
(Dorman's):				
Light	1 oz.	5.0		
Lo-chol	1 oz.	7.0		
Low-sodium	1 oz.	9.0		
(Land O'Lakes)	1 oz.	9.0	5.0	<3.0
Neufchâtel, natural (USDA)	2⅞″ × 2″ × ⅞″ pkg. (3 oz.)	20.4		
Parmesan:				
(USDA) natural:				
Regular	1 oz.	7.4	4.0	3.0
Grated	1 oz.	9.4		
(Progresso) grated	1 T.	2.0	1.0	<1.0
Pot (Sargento)	1 oz.	0.0		
Provolone:				
(Dorman's) light	1 oz.	4.0		
(Land O'Lakes)	1 oz.	8.0	5.0	<3.0
Ricotta:				
(USDA):				
Natural	1 oz.	3.7		
Part skim, natural	1 oz.	4.0		
(Polly-O):				
Lite	1 oz.	2.0		
Old-fashioned	1 oz.	4.0		
Part skim milk, regular or no salt added	1 oz.	3.0		
Whole milk, regular or no salt added		3.5		
Romano:				
(Polly-O) grated	1 oz.	10.0		
(Progresso) grated	1 T.	2.0	1.0	<1.0
Roquefort, natural (USDA)	1 oz.	8.6	4.0	4.0
Samsoe (Sargento) Danish	1 oz.	8.0		
Semi-soft:				
Bel Paese	1 oz.	7.4		

FOOD DESCRIPTION	MEASURE OR QUANTITY	FATS IN GRAMS		
		Total	Saturated	Unsaturated
Laughing Cow:				
Babybel:				
Regular	1 oz.	7.0		
Mini	¾ oz.	6.2		
Bonbel:				
Regular	1 oz.	8.2		
Reduced-calorie	1 oz.	2.5		
Swiss:				
(USDA):				
Natural	1 oz.	7.9	4.0	4.0
Natural	1″ cube (.5 oz.)	4.2	2.0	2.0
Process:				
Regular or reduced sodium	1-oz. slice	7.6	4.0	3.0
Regular or reduced sodium	1″ cube (.6 oz.)	4.8	3.0	2.0
Churny Lite	1 oz.	5.0	3.0	0.0
Taco (Sargento) shredded	1 oz.	9.0		
CHEESE CAKE (See **CAKE,** Cheese)				
CHEESE DIP (See **DIP**)				
CHEESE FONDUE, home recipe (USDA)	4 oz.	20.8	10.0	10.0
CHEESE FOOD, processed:				
American or cheddar:				
(USDA)	1-oz. slice (3½″ × 33/8″ × ⅛″)	6.8	4.0	3.0
(USDA)	1″ cube (.6 oz.)	4.3	2.0	2.0
Heart Beat (GFA) American or sharp	¾-oz. slice	2.0	1.0	0.0
(Land O'Lakes)	¾-oz. slice	5.0	3.0	< .2
(Shedd's) Country Crock, cheddar, any flavor	1 oz.	4.0		
Garlic & herbs, *Wispride*	1 oz.	7.0		
Italian herb (Land O'Lakes)	1 oz.	7.0	4.0	<3.0
Jalapeño (Land O'Lakes)	1 oz.	7.0	4.0	<3.0
Low-sodium, *Heart Beat* (GFA)	.7-oz. slice	2.0	<1.0	0.0
Neufchâtel (Shedd's) Country Crock, any flavor	1 oz.	7.0		
Onion (Land O'Lakes)	1 oz.	7.0	4.0	<3.0
Pepperoni (Land O'Lakes)	1 oz.	7.0	4.0	<3.0
Pizza-Mate (Fisher's)	1 oz.	7.0		
Salami (Land O'Lakes)	1 oz.	7.0	4.0	<3.0
CHEESE SPREAD:				
American, process:				
(USDA) regular or reduced sodium	1 oz.	6.1		
(Nabisco) *Easy Cheese*	1 tsp. (5 grams)	1.0		
Bleu, *Laughing Cow*	1 oz.	6.0		
Cheddar:				
Laughing Cow	1 oz.	6.0		
(Nabisco) *Easy Cheese:*				
Regular or sharp	1 tsp. (.2 oz.)	1.2		
Chive	1 tsp. (.2 oz.)	1.1		
Cheese & bacon (Nabisco) *Easy Cheese*	1 oz.	4.5		
Cheez Whiz, process (Kraft)	1 oz.	4.5		
Golden Velvet (Land O'Lakes)	1 oz.	6.0	4.0	<3.0
Gruyere, *Laughing Cow, La Vache Qui Rit:*				
Regular	1 oz.	6.0		
Reduced calorie	1 oz.	2.6		
Nacho (Nabisco) *Easy Cheese*	1 tsp. (.2 oz.)	1.2		
Pimento (Prince's)	1 oz.	6.0		
Provolone, *Laughing Cow*	1 oz.	6.0		
Velveeta (Kraft) regular	1 oz.	5.0		

FOOD DESCRIPTION	MEASURE OR QUANTITY	FATS IN GRAMS		
		Total	Saturated	Unsaturated
CHEESE STRAW (USDA):				
Made with lard or vegetable shortening	1 oz.	8.5	4.0	5.0
Made with lard or vegetable shortening	5″ × ⅜″ × ⅜″ piece (6 grams)	1.8	<1.0	1.0
CHELOIS WINE (Great Western) 12.5% alcohol	3 fl. oz.	0.0		
CHERRY:				
Sour:				
Fresh (USDA):				
Whole	1 lb. (weighed without stems)	1.3		
Pitted	½ cup (2.7 oz.)	.2		
Canned, syrup pack, pitted:				
(USDA) light, heavy or extra-heavy syrup	4 oz. (with liq.)	.2		
(Thank You Brand)	½ cup (4.5 oz.)	0.0		
Canned, water pack, pitted, solids & liq.:				
(USDA)	½ cup (4.3 oz.)	.2		
(Thank You Brand)	½ cup (4.9 oz.)	0.0		
Frozen, pitted (USDA) sweetened or unsweetened	4 oz.	.5		
Sweet:				
Fresh (USDA):				
Whole, with stems	1 lb. (weighed with stems)	1.2		
Pitted	½ cup (2.9 oz.)	.2		
Canned, syrup pack, with pits, solids & liq.:				
(USDA) light, heavy or extra heavy syrup	4 oz.	.2		
(Del Monte) heavy syrup	½ cup (4.3 oz.)	.6		
Canned, syrup pack, pitted, solids & liq.:				
(USDA) light, heavy or extra heavy syrup	4 oz.	.2		
(Del Monte) heavy syrup	½ cup (4.2 oz.)	1.5		
Canned, water pack, with pits, solids & liq.				
(USDA)	4 oz.	.2		
CHERRY, CANDIED (USDA)	1 oz.	.6		
CHERRY DRINK:				
Canned, regular pack:				
Squeezit (General Mills)	6¾-fl.-oz. container	<1.0		
(Smucker's) black	8 fl. oz.	0.0		
*Mix (Funny Face)	6 fl. oz.	0.0		
CHERRY JELLY, sweetened (Home Brand) or dietetic (Featherweight)	1 T.	0.0		
CHERRY, MARASCHINO (USDA)	1 oz. (with liq.)	< .1		
CHERRY PIE FILLING (See **PIE FILLING,** Cherry)				
CHERRY PRESERVE OR JAM:				
Sweetened (Home Brand)	1 T. (.7 oz.)	0.0		
Dietetic or low-calorie (Estee)	1 T.	Tr.		
CHERVIL, raw (USDA)	1 oz.	.3		
CHESTNUT (USDA):				
Fresh, shelled	4 oz.	1.7		
Dried, shelled	4 oz.	4.6		
CHEWING GUM:				
Sweetened:				
Beechies or *Beech-Nut*	1 piece	0.0		
Juicy Fruit or spearmint (Wrigley's)	1 piece	Tr.		
Unsweetened or dietetic (Estee) all flavors	1 piece	< .1		
*Care*Free*	1 piece	0.0		

FOOD DESCRIPTION	MEASURE OR QUANTITY	FATS IN GRAMS		
		Total	Saturated	Unsaturated
CHEX, cereal (Ralston-Purina):				
Bran (See **BRAN BREAKFAST CEREAL**)				
Corn, double, rice or wheat	Any quantity	0.0		
Honey graham	2/3 cup (1 oz.)	1.0		
Oat, honey nut	1/2 cup (1 oz.)	1.0		
CHICKEN (See also **CHICKEN, CANNED**) (USDA):				
Broiler, cooked, meat only	4 oz.	4.3	1.0	3.0
Capon, raw, ready-to-cook	1 lb. (weighed with bones)	70.2	22.0	48.0
Capon, raw, meat with skin	4 oz.	24.9		
Fryer:				
Raw:				
Ready-to-cook	1 lb. (weighed with bone)	15.1	5.0	10.0
Meat & skin	1 lb.	23.1	7.0	16.0
Meat only	1 lb.	12.2	4.0	8.0
Dark meat with skin	1 lb.	28.6	9.0	20.0
Light meat with skin	1 lb.	17.7	5.0	12.0
Dark meat without skin	1 lb.	17.2	5.0	12.0
Light meat without skin	1 lb.	6.8	2.0	5.0
Skin only	4 oz.	19.4	6.0	14.0
Back	1 lb. (weighed with bone)	23.5	8.0	16.0
Breast	1 lb. (weighed with bone)	8.6	3.0	6.0
Leg or drumstick	1 lb. (weighed with bone)	10.6	3.0	8.0
Neck	1 lb. (weighed with bone)	20.5	7.0	14.0
Rib	1 lb. (weighed with bone)	12.5	4.0	8.0
Thigh	1 lb. (weighed with bone)	19.1	6.0	13.0
Wing	1 lb. (weighed with bone)	16.5	5.0	12.0
Fried. A 2½-pound chicken (weighed with bone before cooking) will give you:				
Back[1]	1 back (2.2 oz.)	8.5	3.0	6.0
Breast[1]	1/2 breast (3.3 oz.)	4.9	2.0	3.0
Leg or drumstick[1]	1 leg (2 oz.)	3.8	1.0	3.0
Neck[1]	1 neck (2.1 oz.)	7.3	3.0	5.0
Rib[1]	1 rib (.7 oz.)	2.2	<1.0	2.0
Thigh[1]	1 thigh (2.3 oz.)	5.7	2.0	4.0
Wing[1]	1 wing (1¾ oz.)	4.3	1.0	3.0
Fryer:				
Fried:				
Meat, skin & giblets[1]	4 oz.	13.4	3.0	10.0
Meat & skin[1]	4 oz.	13.5	3.0	10.0
Meat only[1]	4 oz.	8.8	3.0	6.0
Dark meat with skin[1]	4 oz.	15.4	5.0	10.0
Light meat with skin[1]	4 oz.	11.2	4.0	8.0
Dark meat without skin[1]	4 oz.	10.5	3.0	7.0
Light meat without skin[1]	4 oz.	6.9	2.0	5.0
Skin only[1]	1 oz.	8.2	3.0	6.0
Hen & cock:				
Raw:				
Ready-to-cook	1 lb. (weighed with bones)	82.1	26.0	56.0
Meat & skin	1 lb.	85.3	27.0	58.0
Meat only	1 lb.	31.8	10.0	21.0
Dark meat without skin	1 lb.	34.0	11.0	23.0
Light meat without skin	1 lb.	16.8	5.0	11.0
Stewed:				
Meat, skin & giblets	4 oz.	25.2	8.0	17.0
Meat & skin	4 oz.	25.9	8.0	18.0
Meat only	4 oz.	10.1	3.0	7.0
Chopped	1/2 cup (2.5 oz.)	6.4	2.0	4.0
Diced	1/2 cup (2.4 oz.)	6.0	2.0	4.0
Ground	1/2 cup (2 oz.)	5.0	2.0	3.0
Roaster:				
Raw:				
Ready-to-cook	1 lb. (weighed with bones)	59.3	19.0	40.0
Meat, skin & giblets	1 lb.	54.0	18.0	36.0
Meat & skin	1 lb.	57.2	19.0	38.0

[1]Principal source of fat: vegetable shortening.

FOOD DESCRIPTION	MEASURE OR QUANTITY	FATS IN GRAMS		
		Total	Saturated	Unsaturated
Meat only	1 lb.	20.4	7.0	14.0
Dark meat without skin	1 lb.	21.3	7.0	14.0
White meat without skin	1 lb.	14.5	5.0	10.0
Roasted:				
Total edible	4 oz.	22.9	7.0	16.0
Meat, skin & giblets	4 oz.	15.9	5.0	11.0
Meat & skin	4 oz.	16.7	5.0	11.0
Meat only	4 oz.	7.1	2.0	5.0
Dark meat without skin	4 oz.	7.4	2.0	5.0
Light meat without skin	4 oz.	5.6	2.0	3.0
CHICKEN A LA KING:				
Home recipe (USDA)	1 cup (8.6 oz.)	34.3	12.0	22.0
Canned (Swanson)	5¼-oz. serving	12.0		
Frozen:				
(Armour):				
Classics Lite	11¼-oz. pkg.	7.0		
Dining Lite, & rice	9-oz. pkg.	7.0		
(Stouffer's) with rice	9½-oz. pkg.	9.0		
(Weight Watchers)	9-oz. pkg.	8.0	2.0	6.0
CHICKEN BOUILLION/ BROTH, cube or powder (See also **CHICKEN SOUP**):				
Regular:				
(Herb-Ox) cube or packet	1 cube or 1 packet	.1		
*(Knorr)	8 fl. oz.	1.1		
(Maggi)	1 cube	0.0		
Low-sodium:				
(Borden's) *Lite-Lite*, imitation	1 tsp.	Tr.		
(Featherweight)	1 tsp.	1.0		
CHICKEN, CANNED, BONED:				
(USDA)	½ cup (3 oz.)	9.9	3.0	
(Featherweight) low-sodium	5-oz. serving	18.0		
(Hormel) chunk style:				
Breast	6¾-oz. serving	20.0		
Dark	6¾-oz. serving	18.0		
(Swanson) chunk style:				
Regular	2½-oz. serving	3.0		
Mixin' style	2½-oz. serving	8.0		
White	2½-oz. serving	2.0		
CHICKEN CHUNKS, frozen (Country Pride):				
Regular	¼ of 12-oz. pkg.	15.0		
Southern fried	¼ of 12-oz. pkg.	20.0		
CHICKEN DINNER OR ENTREE:				
Canned:				
(Hunt's) *Minute Gourmet* Microwave Entree Maker:				
Barbecue	6.8-oz. serving	4.0		
Cacciatore	8.3-oz. serving	6.0		
Sweet & sour	7.8-oz. serving	Tr.		
(Swanson) & dumplings	7½-oz. serving	12.0		
Frozen:				
(Armour):				
Classics Lite:				
Breast medallions marsala	10½-oz. serving	7.0		
Oriental	10-oz. serving	1.0		
Dining Lite, glazed	9-oz. serving	4.0		
Dinner Classics:				
Mesquite	9½-oz. serving	16.0		
Parmigiana	11½-oz. serving	19.0		
(Banquet):				
Cookin' Bags, & vegetable primavera	4-oz. serving	2.0		
Dinner:				
Regular:				
& dumplings	10-oz. dinner	24.0		
Fried	10-oz. dinner	22.0		

FOOD DESCRIPTION	MEASURE OR QUANTITY	FATS IN GRAMS		
		Total	Saturated	Unsaturated
ExtraHelping:				
Fried	16-oz. dinner	28.0		
Nuggets:				
with barbecue sauce	10-oz. dinner	36.0		
with sweet & sour sauce	10-oz. dinner	34.0		
Family Entree:				
& dumplings	¼ of 28-oz. pkg.	14.0		
& vegetable primavera	¼ of 28-oz. pkg.	3.0		
Platter:				
Boneless:				
Drumsnacker	7-oz. serving	19.0		
Nuggets	6.4-oz. serving	21.0		
Fried, all white	9-oz. serving	22.0		
(Celentano):				
Parmigiana, cutlets	9-oz. pkg.	2.0		
Primavera	11½-oz. pkg.	7.0		
(Chun King):				
Imperial	13-oz. entree	1.0		
Walnut, crunchy	13-oz. entree	5.0		
(Healthy Choice):				
A L'Orange	9½-oz. meal	2.0	Tr.	Tr.
Glazed	8½-oz. meal	3.0	1.0	1.0
Mesquite	10½-oz. meal	2.0	Tr.	Tr.
Parmigiana	11½-oz. meal	3.0	2.0	Tr.
Sweet & sour	11½-oz. meal	2.0	Tr.	Tr.
(Kids Cusine):				
Fried	7¼-oz. meal	22.0		
Nuggets	6¼-oz. meal	19.0		
(La Choy) *Fresh & Lite:*				
Almond, with rice & vegetables	9¾-oz. meal	8.0		
Sweet & sour	10-oz. meal	3.0		
(Stouffer's):				
Regular:				
Cashew, in sauce with rice	9½-oz. meal	16.0		
Creamed	6½-oz. meal	21.0		
Divan	8½-oz. meal	20.0		
Lean Cuisine:				
A l'orange, with almond rice	8-oz. meal	5.0		
Breast, parmesan	10-oz. meal	8.0		
Cacciatore, with vermicelli	10⅞-oz. meal	7.0		
Glazed, with vegetable rice	8½-oz. meal	8.0		
Right Course:				
Italiano, with fettucini	9⅝-oz. meal	8.0		
Tenderloins, in barbecue sauce	8¾-oz. meal	6.0		
(Swanson):				
Regular, 4-compartment, fried:				
Barbecue flavor	9¼-oz. meal	30.0		
Breast portion	10¾-oz. meal	33.0		
Hungry-Man:				
Boneless	17½-oz. dinner	27.0		
Fried:				
Breast portion	11¾-oz. entree	37.0		
Dark portion with whipped potatoes	11-oz. entree	36.0		
Parmesan	20-oz. dinner	51.0		
(Tyson):				
A L'Orange	9½-oz. meal	8.0		
Dijon	8½-oz. meal	17.0		
Francais	9½-oz. meal	14.0		

FOOD DESCRIPTION	MEASURE OR QUANTITY	FATS IN GRAMS		
		Total	Saturated	Unsaturated
Kiev	9¼-oz. meal	33.0		
Parmigiana	10¼-oz. meal	17.0		
(Weight Watchers):				
Cordon bleu, breaded	8-oz. meal	11.0	4.0	6.0
Fettucini	8¼-oz. meal	10.0	3.0	7.0
Imperial	9¼-oz. meal	4.0	1.0	3.0
Sweet & sour tenders	10.2-oz. meal	1.0	Tr.	Tr.
CHICKEN & DUMPLINGS (See **CHICKEN DINNER**)				
CHICKEN FRICASSEE, home recipe (USDA)	1 cup (8.5 oz.)	22.3	7.0	15.0
CHICKEN, FRIED, frozen:				
(Banquet):				
Assorted	32-oz. pkg.	95.0		
Breast portion	11½-oz. pkg.	22.0		
Hot 'n' Spicy	32-oz. pkg.	95.0		
(Country Pride) Southern fried:				
Chunks	¼ of 12-oz. pkg.	20.0		
Patties	¼ of 12-oz. pkg.	15.0		
(Swanson) *Plump & Juicy:*				
Assorted	3¼-oz. serving	17.0		
Breast	4½-oz. serving	21.0		
Cutlets	3½-oz. serving	13.0		
Dipsters or drumlets	3-oz. serving	14.0		
Nibblers	3¼-oz. serving	20.0		
CHICKEN GIBLETS (USDA):				
Capon, raw	2 oz.	8.3		
Fryer, raw	2 oz.	1.8		
Fryer, fried, from a 2½-lb. chicken	1 heart, gizzard & liver (2.1 oz.)	6.7		
Hen & cock, raw	2 oz.	6.6		
Roaster, raw	2 oz.	2.7		
CHICKEN GIZZARD (USDA):				
Raw	2 oz.	1.5		
Simmered	2 oz.	1.9		
CHICKEN & NOODLES:				
Home recipe (USDA)	1 cup (8.5 oz.)	18.5	5.0	14.0
Frozen:				
(Armour):				
Dining Lite	9-oz. meal	7.0		
Dinner Classics	11-oz. meal	7.0		
(Stouffer's) homestyle	10-oz. meal	15.0		
CHICKEN NUGGETS, frozen (See also *HOT BITES* or **CHICKEN DINNER OR ENTREE**):				
(Country Pride)	¼ of 12-oz. pkg.	16.0		
(Empire Kosher Poultry)	¼ of 12-oz. pkg.	8.0		
CHICKEN, PACKAGED:				
(Louis Rich) breast, oven roasted	1-oz. slice	2.0		
(Oscar Mayer) breast:				
Oven roasted	1-oz. slice	.7	.2	.4
Smoked	1-oz. slice	.3	.1	.3
(Weaver):				
Bologna	1 slice	3.7		
Breast, hickory smoked or oven roasted	1 slice	.8		
Roll	1 slice	1.4		
CHICKEN PATTIES, frozen:				
(Country Pride)	¼ of 12-oz. pkg.	16.0		
(Empire Kosher Poultry)	¼ of 12-oz. pkg.	11.0		
CHICKEN PIE:				
Baked, home recipe (USDA)	⅓ of 9″ pie (8.2 oz.)	31.3	12.0	20.0
Frozen:				
(Banquet)	7-oz. pie	36.0		
(Empire Kosher Poultry)	8-oz. pie	21.0		
(Swanson):				
Regular	8-oz. pie	24.0		

FOOD DESCRIPTION	MEASURE OR QUANTITY	FATS IN GRAMS		
		Total	Saturated	Unsaturated
Chunky	10-oz. pie	33.0		
Hungry-Man	16-oz. pie	37.0		
CHICKEN, POTTED (USDA)	1 oz.	5.4		
CHICKEN SALAD OR SPREAD, canned:				
(Carnation) *Spreadables*	¼ of 7½-oz. can	8.8		
(Hormel) regular or Sandwich Makin's	1 oz.	4.0		
(Underwood)	½ of 4¾-oz. can	10.9		
CHICKEN SOUP MIX (See **SOUP, MIX,** Chicken)				
CHICKEN STEW, canned (Swanson)	7⅝ oz. serving	7.0		
CHICK-FIL-A:				
Brownie, fudge, with nuts	2.8-oz. piece	19.1		
Chicken, no bun	3.6-oz. piece	15.1		
Chicken nuggets, 8-pack	4-oz. serving	15.1		
Chicken salad:				
Regular:				
Cup	3.4-oz. serving	28.2		
Plate	11.8-oz. serving	63.5		
Chargrilled golden	10.4-oz. serving	2.1		
Chicken Salad Sandwich:				
Regular, wheat bread	5.7-oz. serving	26.5		
Chargrilled	5½-oz. serving	4.8		
Chicken Sandwich:				
Regular, with bun	5¾-oz. serving	8.5		
Deluxe, with bun:				
Regular	7.45-oz. serving	8.6		
Chargrilled, with lettuce & tomato	7.15-oz. serving	4.9		
Icedream	4½-oz. serving	4.8		
Pie, lemon	4.1-oz. slice	5.1		
Potato, *Waffle Potato Fries*	3-oz. serving	13.5		
Potato Salad	3.8-oz. cup	15.0		
Salad, tossed:				
Plain	4½-oz. serving	.2		
With dressing:				
Honey French	6-oz. serving	24.2		
Italian, lite	6-oz. serving	2.0		
Ranch	6-oz. serving	16.4		
Thousand island	6-oz. serving	21.9		
Soup, hearty, breast of chicken, small	8½-fl.-oz. serving	2.7		
Tea, iced, unsweetened	9 fl. oz.	Tr.		
CHICK PEA OR GARBANZO:				
Dry (USDA)	1 cup (7.1 oz.)	9.6	Tr.	10.0
Canned, regular pack, solids & liq.:				
(Allen)	½ cup	3.0		
(Goya)	½ cup (4 oz.)	2.0		
CHICORY GREENS, raw (USDA) trimmed	4 oz.	.3		
CHILI OR CHILI CON CARNE:				
Canned, beans only:				
(Comstock)	½ cup (4.4 oz.)	0.0		
(Hunt's)	½ cup	<1.0		
Canned, with beans, regular:				
(Gebhardt) hot	½ of 15-oz. can	22.0	8.0	8.0
(Hormel) regular	½ of 15-oz. can	17.0		
JustRite, hot	4-oz. serving	10.0		
(Old El Paso)	1 cup	7.0		
Canned, without beans, dietetic:				
(Estee)	7½-oz. can	28.0		
(Gebhardt)	7½-oz.	32.0		
(Hormel):				
Regular	7½-oz. serving	32.0		
Short Orders	7½-oz. can	27.0		
JustRite	4-oz. serving	11.0		

FOOD DESCRIPTION	MEASURE OR QUANTITY	FATS IN GRAMS		
		Total	Saturated	Unsaturated
Frozen (Stouffer's):				
Regular with beans	8¾-oz. pkg.	10.0		
Right Course, vegetarian	9¾-oz. pkg.	9.0		
*CHILI OR CHILI CON CARNE, Mix, *Manwich, Chili Fixin's*	8-oz. serving	14.0		
CHILI SAUCE:				
(USDA)	½ cup (4.4 oz.)	.4		
(USDA)	1 T. (.5 oz.)	< .1		
(El Molino) green, mild	1 T.	0.0		
(La Victoria) green	1 T.	<1.0		
(Ortega) hot, medium or mild	1 oz.	.1		
CHILI SEASONING MIX:				
*(Durkee)	1 cup	25.0		
(French's) *Chili-O*	⅙ of pkg.	0.0		
(Lawry's)	1.6-oz. pkg.	1.8		
CHIMICHANGA, frozen:				
Marquez (Fred's Frozen Foods):				
Beef, shredded	5-oz. serving	17.0		
Chicken	5-oz. serving	15.0		
(Old El Paso):				
Regular:				
Beef	1 piece	21.0		
Chicken	1 piece	20.0		
Dinner, festive, Beef	11-oz. dinner	21.0		
Entree, Bean & cheese	1 piece	17.0		
CHIPS (See **CRACKERS** for corn chips and **POTATO CHIPS**)				
CHIVES, raw (USDA)	1 oz.	< .1		
CHOCOLATE, BAKING:				
Bitter or unsweetened:				
(USDA)	1 oz.	15.0	9.0	6.0
(USDA) grated	½ cup (2.3 oz.)	35.0	20.0	15.0
(Baker's)	1-oz. sq.	15.0		
Sweetened:				
Bittersweet (USDA)	1 oz.	11.3	7.0	5.0
Chips, milk (Hershey's)	1 oz.	8.0		
Chips, semisweet (Baker's)	¼ cup (1.5 oz.)	10.5		
Chips, semisweet (Hershey's)	1 oz.	8.0		
German's, sweet (Baker's)	4½″ sq. (1 oz.)	9.3		
Morsels, milk (Nestlé)	1 oz.	9.0		
Morsels, semisweet (Nestlé)	1 oz.	8.0		
Semisweet, small pieces (USDA)	½ cup (3 oz.)	30.3	17.0	13.0
CHOCOLATE CAKE (See **CAKE,** Chocolate)				
CHOCOLATE CANDY (See **CANDY**)				
CHOCOLATE, HOT, home recipe (USDA)	1 cup (8.8 oz.)	12.5	8.0	5.0
CHOCOLATE ICE CREAM (See **ICE CREAM,** Chocolate)				
CHOCOLATE PIE (See **PIE,** Chocolate)				
CHOCOLATE PUDDING (See **PUDDING** or **PIE FILLING,** Chocolate)				
CHOP SUEY:				
Home recipe, with meat (USDA)	1 cup (8.8 oz.)	17.0	7.0	10.0
Frozen:				
(Banquet) beef:				
Buffet Supper	32-oz. pkg.	11.8		
Dinner	12-oz. pkg.	8.2		
(Stouffer's) beef, with rice	12-oz. pkg.	10.0		

FOOD DESCRIPTION	MEASURE OR QUANTITY	FATS IN GRAMS		
		Total	Saturated	Unsaturated
*CHOP SUEY SEASONING MIX (Durkee)	1¾ cups	32.4		
CHOW CHOW (USDA):				
Sour	1 oz.	.4		
Sweet	1 oz.	.3		
CHOW MEIN:				
Home recipe, chicken, without noodles (USDA)	4 oz.	4.5		
Canned:				
(Chun King) Divider-Pak:				
Chicken	¼ of pkg.	3.6		
Shrimp	¼ of pkg.	2.1		
(La Choy):				
Regular:				
Beef, meatless or shrimp	¾ cup	1.0		
Chicken	¾ cup	2.0		
*Bi-pack:				
Beef or shrimp	¾ cup	1.0		
Chicken	¾ cup	3.0		
Frozen:				
(Armour) *Dining Lite*	9-oz. pkg.	2.0		
(Chun King) chicken	13-oz. meal	6.0		
(Empire Kosher) chicken	½ of 15-oz. pkg.	2.0		
(Healthy Choice) chicken	8½-oz. meal	3.0	1.0	1.0
(La Choy):				
Regular:				
Chicken:				
Dinner	12-oz. dinner	4.0		
Entree	⅔ cup	2.0		
Shrimp, dinner	12-oz. dinner	1.0		
Fresh & Lite, imperial, chicken	11-oz. meal	7.0		
(Stouffer's) chicken:				
Regular, without noodles	8-oz. serving	4.0		
Lean Cuisine, with rice	11¼-oz. serving	5.0		
CHOW MEIN NOODLES (See NOODLES, CHOW MEIN)				
CHOW MEIN SEASONING MIX (Kikkoman)	1⅛-oz. pkg.	.8		
CHUB, raw (USDA) meat only	4 oz.	10.0		
CHURCH'S FRIED CHICKEN:				
Chicken, fried:				
Breast	4.3 oz.	17.3		
Leg	2.9 oz.	8.6		
Wing-breast	4.8 oz.	19.7		
Corn, with butter oil	1 ear	9.3		
French fries	1 regular order	5.5		
CIDER (See APPLE CIDER)				
CINNAMON, ground (Information supplied by General Mills Laboratory)	1 oz.	1.0		
CINNAMON TOAST CRUNCH, cereal (General Mills)	¾ cup (1 oz.)	3.0		
CITRON, CANDIED (USDA)	1 oz.	< .1		
CLAM:				
Raw, all kinds, meat only (USDA)	4 med. clams (3 oz.)	1.4		
Raw, hard or round (USDA):				
Meat & liq.	1 lb. (weighed in shell)	.6		
Meat only	1 cup (7 round chowders, 8 oz.)	2.0		
Raw, soft (USDA) meat only	1 cup (19 large, 8 oz.)	4.3		
Canned, all kinds:				
Solids & liq. (USDA)	4 oz.	.8		
Meat only (USDA)	½ cup (2.8 oz.)	2.0		
Minced, drained solids (Gorton's)	1 can	2.0		

FOOD DESCRIPTION	MEASURE OR QUANTITY	FATS IN GRAMS		
		Total	Saturated	Unsaturated
Frozen, fried:				
Strips, crunchy (Gorton's)	3½ oz.	22.0		
Light (Mrs. Paul's)	5-oz. pkg.	26.0		
CLAMATO, cocktail (Mott's)	6 fl. oz.	0.0		
CLAM CHOWDER (See **SOUP,** Chowder, Clam)				
CLARET WINE	Any quantity	0.0		
CLUSTERS, cereal (General Mills)	½ cup (1 oz.)	3.0		
COBBLER, frozen (Pet-Ritz):				
Apple or strawberry	½ cup (1 oz.)	3.0		
Blueberry	⅙ of 26-oz. pkg.	12.0		
COCOA, dry:				
Plain (USDA):				
Low-fat	1 T. (5 grams)	.4	Tr.	Tr.
Medium-low fat	1 T. (5 grams)	.7	Tr.	Tr.
Medium-high fat	½ cup (1.5 oz.)	8.2	5.0	3.0
Medium-high fat	1 T. (5 grams)	1.0	<1.0	Tr.
High-fat	½ cup (1.5 oz.)	10.2	6.0	5.0
Processed with alkali (USDA):				
Medium-low fat	1 T. (5 grams)	.7	Tr.	Tr.
Medium-high fat	1 T. (5 grams)	1.0	<1.0	Tr.
High-fat	1 T. (5 grams)	1.3	<1.0	<1.0
COCOA MIX:				
Regular:				
(Carnation) chocolate with mini-marshmallow, milk chocolate or rich chocolate	1-oz. packet	1.0		
(Hershey's) instant	1 T.	.3		
(Nestlé)	1¼-oz.	4.0		
(Swiss Miss):				
Regular, double rich	1 envelope	3.0		
European creme:				
Amaretto, creme de menthe or mocha	1¼-oz. envelope	4.0		
Chocolate	1¼-oz. envelope	3.0		
Dietetic:				
*(Estee)	6 fl. oz.	Tr.		
(Swiss Miss)	1 envelope	Tr.		
(Weight Watchers)	1 envelope	0.0		
COCOA PUFFS, cereal (General Mills)	1 cup (1 oz.)	1.0		
COCONUT:				
Fresh (USDA):				
Whole	1 lb. (weighed in shell)	83.3	72.0	11.0
Meat only	4 oz.	40.0	34.0	6.0
Grated or shredded	1 firmly packed cup (4.6 oz.)	45.9	39.0	7.0
Grated	1 lightly packed cup (2.9 oz.)	28.2	24.0	4.0
Cream, liq. expressed from grated coconut	4 oz.	36.5	32.0	5.0
Milk, liq. expressed from mixture of grated coconut & water	4 oz.	28.2	24.0	4.0
Water, liq. from coconut	1 cup (8.5 oz.)	.5		
Dried, canned or packaged:				
Sweetened, shredded (USDA)	½ lightly packed cup (1.6 oz.)	18.0	16.0	2.0
Unsweetened (USDA)	½ lightly packed cup (1.6 oz.)	30.0	26.0	4.0
Angel-Flake (Baker's)	½ cup (1.3 oz.)	11.8		
Premium shred (Baker's)	½ cup (⅕ oz.)	13.8		
COCONUT, CREAM OF, canned:				
(Coco Lopez)	1 T.	2.5		
(Holland House)	1 oz.	0.0		
COCO WHEATS, cereal	2 T. (.6 oz.)	.6		

FOOD DESCRIPTION	MEASURE OR QUANTITY	FATS IN GRAMS		
		Total	Saturated	Unsaturated
COD:				
Raw, meat only (USDA)	4 oz.	.3		
Broiled (USDA)	4 oz.	6.0		
Canned (USDA)	4 oz.	.3		
Dried, salted (USDA)	4 oz.	.8		
Frozen (Gorton's)	4 oz.	1.0		
COD DINNER OR ENTREE, frozen (Frionor) *Norway Gourmet:*				
With dill sauce	4.5-oz. piece	0.0		
With toasted bread crumbs	4.5-oz. piece	8.0		
COD LIVER OIL (Hain)	1 T.	14.0		
COFFEE (All coffee, regardless of brand name or type, is essentially the same)	1 cup	Tr.		
COLA SOFT DRINK (See **SOFT DRINK,** Cola)				
COLESLAW, not drained (USDA):				
Prepared with commercial French dressing	4 oz.	8.3	1.0	7.0
Prepared with homemade French dressing, using corn oil	4 oz.	13.9	1.0	13.0
Prepared with mayonnaise	4 oz.	15.9	2.0	14.0
Prepared with mayonnaise-type salad dressing	4 oz.	9.0	1.0	8.0
COLLARDS:				
Raw (USDA) leaves only	½ lb.	1.2		
Boiled without salt, drained (USDA) leaves	½ cup (3.4 oz.)	.7		
Canned, chopped, solids & liq.:				
(Allen)	½ cup (4 oz.)	Tr.		
(Sunshine)	½ cup (4.1 oz.)	.4		
Frozen:				
(Birds Eye) chopped	⅓ of 10-oz. pkg.	.4		
(Frosty Acres)	⅓ of 10-oz. pkg.	0.0		
CONCORD WINE	Any quantity	0.0		
COOKIE, COMMERCIAL:				
Almond Supreme (Pepperidge Farm)	1 piece	5.0		
Almond toast (Stella D'Oro)	1 piece	1.0		
Angelica Goodies (Stella D'Oro)	1 piece	4.0		
Angel Wings (Stella D'Oro)	1 piece	5.0		
Anginette (Stella D'Oro)	1 piece	1.0		
Animal:				
(FFV)	1 piece	.4	.1	.1
(Nabisco) *Barnum's Animals*	1 piece	.4		
(Tom's)	½ oz.	5.0		
Anisette sponge (Stella D'Oro)	1 piece	1.0		
Anisette toast (Stella D'Oro)	1 piece	1.0		
Apple N' Raisin (Archway)	1 piece	3.0		
Assortment:				
(Nabisco) *Mayfair:*				
Crown creme sandwich	1 piece	2.3		
Fancy shortbread biscuit	1 piece	1.7		
Mayfair creme sandwich	1 piece	3.0		
(Pepperidge Farm):				
Butter or *Seville*	1 piece	3.0		
Champagne	1 piece	1.3		
Southport	1 piece	4.5		
Blueberry Newtons (Nabisco)	1 piece	1.3		
Bordeaux (Pepperidge Farm)	1 piece	1.6		
Breakfast Treats (Stella D'Oro)	1 piece	4.0		
Brown edge wafer (Nabisco)	1 piece	1.5		

FOOD DESCRIPTION	MEASURE OR QUANTITY	FATS IN GRAMS		
		Total	Saturated	Unsaturated
Brownie:				
(Nabisco) *Almost Home*	1¼-oz. piece	7.0		
(Weight Watchers) frozen	1¼-oz. serving	3.0	1.0	3.0
Brussels (Pepperidge Farm)	1 piece	2.6		
Butter (Sunshine)	1 piece	1.0		
Cappucino (Pepperidge Farm)	1 piece	3.0		
Caramel Patties (FFV)	1 piece	3.5		
Castelets (Stella D'Oro) regular or chocolate	1 piece	3.0		
Chessman (Pepperidge Farm)	1 piece	2.0		
Chocolate & chocolate covered:				
(Keebler) stripes	1 piece	3.0		
(Nabisco):				
Pin Wheel, cake	1 piece	5.0		
Snaps	1 piece	.6		
Chocolate chip:				
(Archway) & toffee	1 piece	7.0		
(Keebler) *Rich 'n Chips*	1 piece	4.0		
(Nabisco):				
Almost Home, fudge	1 piece	2.5		
Chips Ahoy:				
Regular	1 piece	2.3		
Chewy	1 piece	3.0		
(Pepperidge Farm) regular	1 piece	2.6		
(Sunshine):				
Chip-A-Roos, regular	1 piece	3.0		
Chippy Chews	1 piece	2.0		
Como Delights (Stella D'Oro)	1 piece	7.0		
Danish (Nabisco) imported	1 piece	1.6		
Dinosaurs (FFV)	1 piece	4.0		
Egg biscuit (Stella D'Oro) sugared:				
Regular	1 piece	1.0		
Roman	1 piece	5.0		
Egg jumbo (Stella D'Oro)	1 piece	1.0		
Fig bar:				
(FFV):				
Vanilla	1 piece	1.0	< 1.0	< 1.0
Whole wheat	1 piece	2.0	< 1.0	< 1.0
(Nabisco) *Fig Newtons*	1 piece	1.0		
(Tom's)	1.8-oz. serving	2.0		
Fruit slices (Stella D'Oro)	1 piece	2.0		
Fruit Stick (Nabisco) *Almost Home:*				
Apple	1 piece	2.5		
Blueberry or cherry	1 piece	2.0		
Fudge (Stella D'Oro):				
Regular	1 piece	2.0		
Deep night	1 piece	4.0		
Swiss	1 piece	3.0		
Gingerman (Pepperidge Farm)	1 piece	1.3		
Ginger Snap:				
(Archway)	1 piece	< 1.0		
(FFV)	1 oz.	4.0		
(Sunshine)	1 piece	.7		
Golden bar (Stella D'Oro)	1 piece	4.0		
Golden Fruit Raisin (Sunshine)	1 piece	.7		
Holiday Trinkets (Stella D'Oro)	1 piece	2.0		
Ladyfinger (USDA)	3¼″ × 1⅜″ × 1⅛″	.9	.2	.7
Lido (Pepperidge Farm)	1 piece	.5		
Love (Stella D'Oro)	1 piece	5.0		
Macaroon:				
(Archway) coconut	1 piece	3.0		
(Nabisco) soft	1 piece	9.0		
(Stella D'Oro) coconut	1 piece	3.0		

FOOD DESCRIPTION	MEASURE OR QUANTITY	FATS IN GRAMS		
		Total	Saturated	Unsaturated
Mallopuffs (Sunshine)	1 piece	2.0		
Margherite (Stella D'Oro) chocolate or vanilla	1 piece	3.0		
Marshmallow: (Nabisco):				
Mallomars	1 piece	3.0		
Puffs, cocoa covered	1 piece	4.0		
Milano (Pepperidge Farm)	1 piece	3.3		
Mint Milano (Pepperidge Farm)	1 piece	4.3		
Molasses Crisp (Pepperidge Farm)	1 piece	1.6		
Oatmeal: (Archway):				
Regular, apple bran, raisin or raisin bran	1 piece	3.0		
Apple filled	1 piece	1.0		
Golden, *Ruth's*	1 piece	4.0		
(FFV):				
Regular	1 piece	.8		
Bar, any flavor	1 piece	2.0	< 1.0	< 1.0
(Keebler) old-fashioned	1 piece	3.0		
(Nabisco) *Bakers Bonus*	1 piece	2.5		
(Pepperidge Farm) Irish	1 piece	2.3		
Orange Milano (Pepperidge Farm)	1 piece	4.3		
Peach Apricot bar (FFV):				
Vanilla	1 piece	1.0	< 1.0	< 1.0
Whole wheat	1 piece	2.0	< 1.0	< 1.0
Peanut & peanut butter (Nabisco) *Almost Home,* regular	1 piece	3.5		
Pferrernusse (Stella D'Oro) spice drops	1 piece	1.0		
Raisin: (Nabisco) *Almost Home:*				
Fudge chocolate chip	1 piece	2.5		
Iced applesauce	1 piece	4.0		
(Pepperidge Farm) bran	1 piece	2.7		
Raisin bran (Pepperidge Farm) *Kitchen Hearth*	1 piece	2.7		
Rocky road (Archway)	1 piece	6.0		
Royal Kreem Pilot Bread (FFV)	1 piece	2.0		
Sandwich:				
(FFV) mint	1 piece	3.5		
(Keebler) *Pitter Patter*	1 piece	4.0		
(Nabisco):				
Regular:				
Baronet	1 piece	2.0		
I Screams	1 piece	3.5		
Oreo, regular	1 piece	2.0		
Almost Home, fudge	1 piece	6.0		
(Sunshine):				
Regular, *Hydrox*	1 piece	2.0		
Tru-Blu	1 piece	3.0		
Shortbread or shortcake: (FFV):				
Country	1 piece	4.0		
Striped, *Double Pleasure*	1 piece	3.0		
(Nabisco):				
Lorna Doone	1 piece	1.7		
Pecan	1 piece	4.5		
Social Tea, biscuit (Nabisco)	1 piece	.7		
Strawberry filled (Archway)	1 piece	3.0		
Sugar wafer:				
(Nabisco) *Biscos*	1 piece	.9		
(Sunshine)	1 piece	2.0		
Toy (Sunshine)	1 piece	.4		

FOOD DESCRIPTION	MEASURE OR QUANTITY	FATS IN GRAMS		
		Total	**Saturated**	**Unsaturated**
Vanilla wafer:				
(FFV)	1 piece	.6	Tr.	Tr.
(Sunshine)	1 piece	1.0		
COOKIE CRISP, cereal, chocolate chip or vanilla	1 cup (1 oz.)	1.1		
COOKIE, DIETETIC:				
Almond chocolate wafer (Estee)	1 piece	1.7		
Angel puffs (Stella D'Oro)	1 piece (3 grams)	1.0		
Apple pastry (Stella D'Oro)	1 piece (.8 oz.)	3.9		
Assorted (Estee)	1 piece (6 grams)	1.4	Tr.	1.0
Belgium Treats (Estee)	1 piece	1.7		
Chocolate chip (Estee)	1 piece (6 grams)	1.0	Tr.	< 1.0
Chocolate & vanilla wafer (Estee)	1 piece (4 grams)	1.3	Tr.	1.0
Egg biscuit	1 piece	1.0		
Fig pastry (Stella D'Oro)	1 piece (.9 oz.)	3.7		
Have-a-Heart (Stella D'Oro)	1 piece (.7 oz.)	5.1		
Holland bittersweet wafer (Estee)	1 piece	8.3		
Holland milk chocolate wafer (Estee)	1 piece (.8 oz.)	8.3	3.0	6.0
Kichel (Stella D'Oro)	1 piece (1 gram)	.5		
Oatmeal raisin (Estee)	1 piece (7 grams)	1.4	Tr.	1.0
Prune pastry (Stella D'Oro)	1 piece (.8 oz.)	3.4		
Royal Nuggets (Stella D'Oro)	1 piece (< 1 gram)	.1		
COOKIE DOUGH:				
*Refrigerated (Pillsbury):				
Brownie, fudge, microwave, with chocolate-flavored chips	1/9 of pkg.	9.0		
Chocolate chip, chocolate chocolate chip, oatmeal raisin, peanut butter or sugar	1 cookie	3.0	< 1.0	< 1.0
*Frozen (Rich's):				
Chocolate chip	1 cookie	5.9		
Oatmeal:				
Regular	1 cookie	5.2		
With raisins	1 cookie	4.4		
Peanut butter	1 cookie	6.5		
Sugar	1 cookie	5.4		
COOKIE, HOME RECIPE				
(USDA):				
Brownie with nuts:				
Made with butter	1 oz.	8.5	3.0	6.0
Made with vegetable shortening	1 oz.	8.9	2.0	7.0
Chocolate Chip:				
Made with butter	1 oz.	8.0	4.0	4.0
Made with vegetable shortening	1 oz.	8.5	2.0	6.0
Sugar, soft, thick, made with butter	1 oz.	4.3	2.0	2.0
COOKIE MIX:				
Plain, dry (USDA)	1 oz.	6.9	2.0	5.0
Brownie:				
*(Betty Crocker):				
Caramel swirl	1/24 of pkg.	4.0	1.0	3.0
Chocolate chip or frosted	1/24 of pkg.	6.0	2.0	4.0
Fudge:				
Regular size	1/16 of pkg.	6.0	2.0	4.0
Supreme	1/24 of pkg.	3.0	1.0	< 3.0
German chocolate or walnut	1/24 of pkg.	7.0	1.0	6.0
(Duncan Hines):				
Chewy recipe	1/24 of pkg.	2.3		
Fudge, original	1/24 of pkg.	2.8		
Peanut butter	1/24 of pkg.	4.8		

FOOD DESCRIPTION	MEASURE OR QUANTITY	FATS IN GRAMS		
		Total	Saturated	Unsaturated
*(Pillsbury) fudge:				
Deluxe:				
Plain	2" square (1/16 pkg.)	6.0		
With walnuts	2" square (1/16 pkg.)	8.0		
Microwave	1/9 of pkg.	9.0		
Ultimate:				
Caramel fudge chunk	2" square (1/6 pkg.)	7.0		
Rocky road	2" square (1/16 pkg.)	8.0		
Chocolate chip:				
*(Betty Crocker) Big Batch	1 cookie	3.0		
(Duncan Hines)	1/36 of pkg.	3.7		
*Date bar (Betty Crocker)	1/24 of pkg.	2.0		
Oatmeal:				
(Duncan Hines) raisin	1/36 of pkg.	3.1		
*(Quaker)	1 cookie	2.8		
Peanut butter (Duncan Hines)	1/36 of pkg.	3.1		
COOKING SPRAY:				
Mazola No Stick	2½-second spray	.7	.1	.5
(Weight Watchers)	1-second spray	1.0		
CORN:				
Fresh, white or yellow (USDA):				
Raw, trimmed, on cob	1 lb. (husk removed)	2.5		
Raw, kernels	4 oz.	1.1		
Boiled without salt, kernels, cut from cob, drained	1 cup (5.9 oz.)	1.7		
Canned, regular pack:				
(Comstock) solids and liq., whole kernel or cream style	½ cup	0.0		
(Green Giant) solids and liq.:				
Cream style	½ of 8½-oz. can	1.0		
Whole kernel:				
Regular or shoepeg	¼ of 17-oz. can	1.0		
Mexicorn	½ of 7-oz. can	Tr.		
Vacuum pack	½ of 7-oz. can	0.0		
(Larsen) *Freshlike,* solids and liq., any style	½ cup	1.0		
Canned, white or yellow, dietetic pack:				
(Diet Delight) whole kernel, solids & liq.	½ cup (4.4 oz.)	0.0		
(Larsen) *Fresh-Lite,* whole kernel, water pack, solids & liq.	½ cup (4.5 oz.)	1.0		
Frozen:				
(Birds Eye):				
On the cob:				
Farmside	4.4-oz. ear	1.0		
Little Ears	2.3-oz. ear	.5		
Whole kernel:				
Plain	1/3 of 10-oz. pkg.	.7		
With butter sauce	1/3 of 10-oz. pkg.	1.0		
(Frosty Acres):				
On the cob	1 whole ear	.5		
Kernels	3.3 oz.	1.0		
(Green Giant):				
On the cob, *Nibblers*	2.7-oz. ear	1.0		
Whole kernel:				
In cream sauce, *Niblets*	½ cup	5.0		
Polybag, *Niblets*	½ cup	1.0		
Shoepeg, white, in butter sauce	½ cup	2.0		
(Larsen) on the cob	3" or 5" piece	1.0		
(Ore-Ida) cob corn	5.3-oz. ear	1.0	< 1.0	< 1.0
CORNBREAD:				
Corn pone, home recipe, prepared with white, whole-ground cornmeal (USDA)	4 oz.	6.0	2.0	4.0

FOOD DESCRIPTION	MEASURE OR QUANTITY	FATS IN GRAMS Total	Saturated	Unsaturated
Johnnycake, home recipe, prepared with yellow, degermed cornmeal (USDA)	4 oz.	5.9	2.0	4.0
Southern-style, home recipe, prepared with degermed cornmeal (USDA)	2½" × 2½" × 1⅝" piece (2.9 oz.)	5.0	1.0	4.0
Southern-style, home recipe, prepared with whole-ground cornmeal (USDA)	4 oz.	8.2	2.0	6.0
Spoonbread, home recipe, prepared with white, whole-ground cornmeal (USDA)	4 oz.	12.9	5.0	8.0
CORNBREAD MIX:				
*Prepared with egg & milk:				
(USDA)	2⅜" muffin (1.4 oz.)	3.4	1.0	2.0
(USDA)	2½" × 2½" × 1⅜" piece (1.9 oz.)	4.6	2.0	3.0
*(Dromedary)	2" × 2" piece (1.4 oz.)	3.0		
**Gold Medal*, white or yellow	⅙ of pkg.	5.0		
CORN DOG, frozen *Little Juan* (Fred's Frozen Foods)	2¾-oz. serving	11.6		
CORNED BEEF:				
Uncooked, boneless, medium fat (USDA)	1 lb.	113.4	54.0	59.0
Cooked, boneless, medium fat (USDA)	4 oz.	34.5	17.0	17.0
Canned:				
(USDA) lean	4 oz.	9.1	5.0	5.0
(Libby's)	⅓ of 7-oz. can	9.0		
Packaged:				
(Carl Buddig)	1 oz.	2.0	.9	.9
(Oscar Mayer)	.6-oz. slice	.3	.2	.2
CORNED BEEF HASH, canned:				
With potato (USDA)	4 oz.	12.8	6.0	7.0
(Libby's)	½ of 15-oz. can	27.0		
Mary Kitchen (Hormel) regular or *Short Orders*	7½-oz. serving	24.0		
CORNED BEEF HASH DINNER, frozen (Banquet)	10-oz. dinner	13.3		
CORNED BEEF SPREAD (Underwood)	4½-oz. can	20.0		
CORN FLAKES, cereal:				
(Featherweight) low-sodium	1¼ cups	0.0		
(General Mills) *Country*	1 cup (1 oz.)	<1.0		
(Kellogg's) regular or sugar-frosted	¾ cup (1 oz.)	0.0		
CORN GRITS (See **HOMINY**)				
CORNMEAL MIX:				
Bolted (Aunt Jemima)	¼ cup (1 oz.)	.7		
Self-rising (Aunt Jemima)	¼ cup (1 oz.)	.9		
CORNMEAL, WHITE OR YELLOW:				
Dry (USDA):				
Bolted or self-rising	1 cup (4.3 oz.)	4.1	Tr.	4.0
Degermed	1 cup (4.3 oz.)	1.7		
Self-rising, degermed	1 cup (5 oz.)	1.6		
Whole-ground, unbolted	1 cup (4.3 oz.)	4.8	Tr.	5.0
Cooked:				
*Bolted (Aunt Jemima)	⅔ cup	.7		
*Degermed (Albers)	1 cup	.5		
*Degermed (Aunt Jemima)	⅔ cup	.3		
CORN POPS, cereal (Kellogg's)	1 cup (1 oz.)	0.0		
CORNSTARCH (Argo)	1 T. (10 grams)	Tr.	Tr.	
CORN *TOTAL*, cereal (General Mills)	1 cup (1 oz.)	1.0		

FOOD DESCRIPTION	MEASURE OR QUANTITY	FATS IN GRAMS		
		Total	Saturated	Unsaturated
COTTAGE PUDDING, home recipe (USDA):				
Without sauce	2 oz.	6.4	4.0	3.0
With chocolate or strawberry sauce	2 oz.	5.0		
COUGH DROP:				
(Estee)	1 drop	Tr.		
(Pine Bros.)	1 drop (3 grams)	0.0		
COUNT CHOCULA, cereal				
(General Mills)	1 cup (1 oz.)	1.0		
COWPEA, including black-eyed peas (USDA):				
Immature seeds:				
Raw, shelled	½ cup (2.5 oz.)	.6		
Boiled, without salt, drained	½ cup (2.9 oz.)	1.7		
Canned, solids & liq.	4 oz.	.3		
Frozen (See **BLACK-EYED PEA,** frozen)				
Young pods with seeds:				
Raw, whole	1 lb. (weighed untrimmed)	1.2		
Boiled without salt, drained	4 oz.	.3		
Mature seeds, dry:				
Raw	½ cup (3 oz.)	1.3		
Boiled without salt, drained	½ cup (4.4 oz.)	.4		
CRAB, all species:				
Fresh (USDA) steamed, meat only	1 cup (4.4 oz.)	2.4		
Canned:				
Drained solids (USDA)	1 packed cup (5.6 oz.)	4.0		
(Del Monte) Alaska king	7½-oz. can	.6		
Frozen (Wakefield's) Alaska king, thawed & drained	4 oz.	1.1		
CRAB APPLE, fresh (USDA) flesh only	4 oz.	.3		
CRAB, DEVILED:				
Home, recipe (USDA)	1 cup (8.5 oz.)	22.6		
Frozen (Mrs. Paul's)	3-oz. piece	6.0		
CRAB, IMITATION (See **SURIMI**)				
CRAB IMPERIAL, home recipe (USDA)	1 cup (7.8 oz.)	16.7		
CRACKERS, PUFFS AND CHIPS:				
Arrowroot biscuit (Nabisco)	1 piece	.7		
Bacon-flavored thins (Nabisco)	1 piece	.6	.3	Tr.
Bugles (Tom's)	1 oz.	8.0		
Cheese flavored:				
American Heritage (Sunshine) cheddar	1 piece	.8		
Chee-Tos, crunchy	1 oz.	10.0		
Cheez Curls (Planters)	1 oz.	11.0		
Cheeze-It (Sunshine)	1 piece	.3		
Nips (Nabisco)	1 piece	.2		
Tid-Bit (Nabisco)	1 piece	.3		
Chicken in a Biskit (Nabisco)	1 piece	.7	.1	Tr.
Club cracker (Keebler)	1 piece	.7		
Corn chips:				
Fritos (Frito-Lay):				
Regular	1 oz.	9.0		
Barbecue flavor	1 oz.	10.0		
Happy Heart (TKI Foods)	⅜ oz.	Tr.		
Heart Lovers (TKI Foods)	⅜ oz.	Tr.		
(Laura Scudder's)	1 oz.	10.0		
Crown Pilot (Nabisco)	1 piece	2.0	Tr.	Tr.
English Water Biscuit (Pepperidge Farm)	1 piece	.4		
Escort (Nabisco)	1 piece	1.3	Tr.	Tr.

FOOD DESCRIPTION	MEASURE OR QUANTITY	FATS IN GRAMS Total	Saturated	Unsaturated
Goldfish (Pepperidge Farm)				
tiny	1 piece	Tr.		
Graham:				
Cinnamon Crisp (Keebler)	1 piece	.5		
(Dixie Belle) sugar-honey coated	1 piece	.4		
(Sunshine) cinnamon	1 piece	.7		
Graham, chocolate- or cocoa-covered:				
(Keebler)	1 piece	2.0		
(Nabisco)	1 piece	2.7		
Great Snackers (Weight Watchers) any flavor	.5-oz. pkg.	3.0		
Hi-Ho (Sunshine)	1 piece	1.2		
Melba Toast (See **MELBA TOAST**)				
Ocean Crisp (FFV)	1 piece	2.0	Tr.	Tr.
Oyster:				
(Nabisco) Dandy or Oysterettes	1 piece	Tr.		
(Sunshine)	1 piece	.1		
Party (Estee)	½ oz.	4.0		
Party mix (Flavor Tree)	1 oz.	11.0		
Pizza Crunchies (Planters)	1 oz.	10.0		
Ritz (Nabisco)	1 piece	1.0	Tr.	Tr.
Ritz Bits (Nabisco):				
Regular, cheese or low-salt	1 piece	.2	Tr.	Tr.
Cheese sandwich	1 piece	.8	.2	Tr.
Peanut butter	1 piece	.7	Tr.	Tr.
Roman Meal Wafer, boxed	1 piece	.5		
Royal Lunch (Nabisco)	1 piece	2.0		
Rye toast (Keebler)	1 piece	.8		
Ry-Krisp:				
Natural	1 triple cracker	0.0		
Seasoned	1 triple cracker	.4		
Sesame	1 triple cracker	1.0		
Saltine:				
(Dixie Belle) regular	1 piece	.3		
Krispy (Sunshine)	1 piece	.2		
Premium (Nabisco) unsalted	1 piece	.4		
Zesta (Keebler)	1 piece	.4		
Sesame:				
American Heritage (Sunshine)	1 piece	1.0		
Chip (Flavor Tree)	1 oz.	10.0		
(Estee)	½ oz.	4.0		
Toast (Keebler)	1 piece	.8		
Snackers (Ralston)	1 piece	.8		
Sociables (Nabisco)	1 piece	.5	Tr.	Tr.
Sour cream-onion stick (Flavor Tree)	1 oz.	10.0		
Table Water Cracker (Carr's) small	1 piece	.7		
Tortilla chips:				
Doritos:				
Regular	1 oz.	6.0		
Cool Ranch:				
Regular	1 oz.	7.0		
Light	1 oz.	4.0		
Salsa Rio	1 oz.	7.0		
Taco	1 oz.	7.0		
(Eagle)				
Nacho, ranch or strips	1 oz.	8.0		
Restaurant style	1 oz.	7.0		
(Old El Paso):				
Crispy corn	1 oz.	8.0		
Nachips	1 oz.	7.0		

FOOD DESCRIPTION	MEASURE OR QUANTITY	FATS IN GRAMS		
		Total	Saturated	Unsaturated
Town House (Keebler's)	1 piece	1.0		
Triscuit (Nabisco):				
Regular, low-salt or wheat & bran	1 piece	.7	Tr.	Tr.
Bits	1 piece	.2	Tr.	Tr.
Twigs (Nabisco)	1 piece	.8	Tr.	Tr.
Uneeda Biscuit (Nabisco) unsalted	1 piece	1.0	Tr.	Tr.
Waverly (Nabisco)	1 piece	.7	Tr.	Tr.
Wheat (Pepperidge Farm) cracked or hearty	1 piece	1.4		
Wheatsworth (Nabisco)	1 piece	Tr.	Tr.	Tr.
Wheat Thins (Nabisco)	1 piece	.4	Tr.	Tr.
CRACKER CRUMBS, GRAHAM:				
(Keebler)	3 oz.	9.9		
(Nabisco)	1½ cups (4.6 oz.) or 9" pie shell	14.0		
CRACKER JACK (See POPCORN)				
CRACKER MEAL:				
(USDA)	3.0 oz.	11.1	3.0	8.0
(USDA)	1 T. (.4 oz.)	1.3	Tr.	1.0
CRANAPPLE (Ocean Spray) canned, regular or low-calorie	6 fl. oz.	Tr.		
CRANBERRY, fresh:				
Untrimmed (USDA)	1 lb. (weighed with stems)	3.0		
(Ocean Spray)	1 oz.	.5		
CRANBERRY JUICE COCKTAIL:				
Canned (Ocean Spray) regular or low-calorie	½ cup (4.4 oz.)	Tr.		
*Frozen (Sunkist)	6 fl. oz.	.1		
CRANBERRY-ORANGE RELISH, canned (Ocean Spray)	4 oz.	.4		
CRANBERRY SAUCE:				
Home recipe, unsweetened, unstrained (USDA)	4 oz.	.3		
Canned:				
Sweetened, strained (USDA)	4 oz.	.3		
(Ocean Spray) jellied or whole berry	4 oz.	.2		
CRAN-FRUIT, cranberry sauce (Ocean Spray) any flavor	2 oz.	Tr.		
CRANGRAPE, juice drink, canned (Ocean Spray)	6 fl. oz.	Tr.		
CRANICOT, juice drink, canned (Ocean Spray)	6 fl. oz.	Tr.		
CRAN-RASPBERRY, juice drink, canned (Ocean Spray) regular or low-calorie	6 fl. oz.	Tr.		
CRANTASTIC, juice drink, canned (Ocean Spray)	6 fl. oz.	Tr.		
CREAM:				
Half & half:				
(USDA)	1 cup (8.5 oz.)	28.2	15.0	14.0
(Johanna)	1 T. (.5 oz.)	1.7		
(Land O'Lakes)	1 T. (.5 oz.)	2.0	1.0	<2.0
Light, table or coffee:				
(USDA)	1 cup (8.5 oz.)	49.4	26.0	23.0
(Johanna Farms) 18% butterfat	1 T. (.5 oz.)	2.9		
Light whipping:				
(USDA)	1 cup (8.4 oz.)	74.8	41.0	34.0
(Sealtest)	1 T. (.5 oz.)	4.5		

FOOD DESCRIPTION	MEASURE OR QUANTITY	FATS IN GRAMS		
		Total	Saturated	Unsaturated
Heavy whipping: (USDA):				
Unwhipped	1 cup (8.4 oz.) or 2 cups whipped	89.5	50.0	40.0
Unwhipped	1 T. (.5 oz.)	5.6	3.0	2.0
(Johanna Farms) 36% butterfat	1 T. (.5 oz.)	5.6		
(Land O'Lakes) gourmet	1 T. (.5 oz.)	5.0	3.0	<3.0
Sour:				
(USDA)	1 cup (8.1 oz.)	47.4	25.0	22.0
(Borden's)	1 T. (.5 oz.)	2.7		
(Sealtest)	1 T. (.5 oz.)	2.7		
CREAM PUFF, home recipe, with custard filling (USDA)	3½" × 2" (4.6 oz.)	18.1	5.0	13.0
CREAM SUBSTITUTE:				
Liquid, frozen (USDA)	1 tsp. (5 grams)	.6	Tr.	Tr.
Powdered (USDA)	1 tsp. (2 grams)	1.0	Tr.	Tr.
Coffee Rich (Rich's)	½ oz.	1.4	.9	.5
Mocha Mix (Presto Food Products)	1 T. (.5 oz.)	1.6	0.0	1.0
CREAM OF WHEAT, cereal	Any quantity	0.0		
CRESS, GARDEN (USDA):				
Raw, whole	1 lb. (weighed untrimmed)	2.3		
Boiled, drained (USDA)	1 cup (6.3 oz.)	1.1		
CRISPIX, cereal (Kellogg's)	¾ cup (1 oz.)	0.0		
CRISP RICE, cereal:				
(Malt-O-Meal) *Crisp 'N Crackling Rice*	1 cup (1 oz.)	.3	.1	
(Ralston-Purina)	1 cup (1 oz.)	.1		
CRISPY WHEATS 'N RAISINS, cereal (General Mills)	¾ cup (1 oz.)	1.0		
CROAKER (USDA):				
Atlantic:				
Raw:				
Meat only	4 oz.	2.5		
Baked	4 oz.	3.6		
White or Yellowfin, raw, meat only	4 oz.	.9		
CROUTON:				
(Kellogg's) *Croutettes*	⅔ cup (.7 oz.)	0.0		
(Pepperidge Farm) any flavor	1/12 of 6-oz. box	3.0		
CUCUMBER, fresh (USDA):				
Eaten with or without skin	½ lb. (weighed with skin)	.2		
Pared	6 slices (2" × ⅛", 1.8 oz.)	Tr.		
CUPCAKE:				
Home recipe (USDA):				
Made with butter, without icing	2¾" cupcake (1.4 oz.)	5.1	3.0	2.0
Made with vegetable shortening, without icing	2¾" cupcake (1.4 oz.)	5.6	2.0	4.0
With chocolate icing	2¾" cupcake (1.8 oz.)	7.0		
With boiled white icing	2¾" cupcake (1.8 oz.)	5.2		
Commercial type (Hostess):				
Chocolate	1¾-oz. piece	4.5		
Orange	1½-oz. piece	4.3		
CUPCAKE MIX:				
*(USDA):				
Prepared with eggs, milk, without icing	2½" cupcake (.9 oz.)	3.0	Tr.	2.0
Prepared with eggs, milk, with chocolate icing	2½" cupcake (1.2 oz.)	4.5	2.0	3.0
*(Flako)	1 large cupcake (1.3 oz., 1/12 of pkg.)	5.0		
CURRANT:				
Fresh (USDA):				
Black European, stems removed	4 oz.	.1		
Red & white, stems removed	4 oz.	.2		
Dried, Zante (Sun-Maid)	½ cup (2.5 oz.)	0.0		

FOOD DESCRIPTION	MEASURE OR QUANTITY	FATS IN GRAMS		
		Total	Saturated	Unsaturated
CURRY POWDER (Crosse & Blackwell)	1 T. (6 grams)	.2		
CUSTARD:				
Home recipe, baked (USDA)	½ cup (4.7 oz.)	7.3	4.0	3.0
Canned (Thank You Brand) egg	½ cup	5.2		
Chilled (Swiss Miss) chocolate or egg	4 oz.	6.0		
CUSTARD, FROZEN (See **ICE CREAM**)				
C.W. POST, cereal (Post) hearty granola	¼ cup (1 oz.)	3.9		
DAIQUIRI COCKTAIL:				
Canned (National Distillers) *Duet,* 12½% alcohol	8 fl.-oz. can	0.0		
Mix (Holland House) liquid or instant	Any quantity	0.0		
*Frozen, mix (Bacardi)	4 fl. oz.	Tr.		
DAIRY QUEEN:				
Banana split	13.5-oz. serving	11.0		
Brownie Delight, hot fudge	9.4-oz. serving	25.0		
Buster Bar	5¼-oz. piece	29.0		
Chicken sandwich	7.8-oz. sandwich	41.0		
Cone:				
Plain, any flavor, regular	5-oz. cone	7.0		
Dipped, chocolate, regular	5½-oz. cone	16.0		
Dilly Bar	3-oz. piece	13.0		
Double Delight	9-oz. serving	20.0		
DQ Sandwich	2.1-oz. sandwich	4.0		
Fish sandwich:				
Plain	6-oz. sandwich	17.0		
With cheese	6¼-oz. sandwich	21.0		
Float	14-oz. serving	7.0		
Freeze, vanilla	12-oz. serving	12.0		
French fries, regular	2½-oz. serving	10.0		
Hamburger:				
Plain:				
Single	5.2-oz. burger	16.0		
Double	7.4-oz. burger	28.0		
With cheese:				
Single	5.7-oz. burger	20.0		
Triple	10.6-oz. burger	50.0		
Hot dog:				
Regular:				
Plain	3½-oz. serving	16.0		
With cheese	4-oz. serving	21.0		
With chili	4½-oz. serving	20.0		
Super:				
Plain	6.2-oz. serving	27.0		
With cheese	6.9-oz. serving	34.0		
With chili	7.7-oz. serving	32.0		
Malt, chocolate:				
Regular	14¾-oz. serving	18.0		
Large	20¾-oz. serving	25.0		
Mr. Misty:				
Plain or Kiss	Any size	0.0		
Float	14½-oz. serving	7.0		
Freeze	14½-oz. serving	12.0		
Onion rings	3-oz. serving	16.0		
Parfait	10-oz. serving	8.0		
Peanut Butter Parfait	10¾-oz. serving	34.0		
Shake, chocolate:				
Small	10¼-oz. serving	13.0		
Regular	14¾-oz. serving	19.0		
Large	20¾-oz. serving	26.0		
Strawberry shortcake	11-oz. serving	11.0		
Sundae, chocolate:				
Small	3¾-oz. serving	4.0		
Regular	6¼-oz. serving	8.0		
Large	8¾-oz. serving	10.0		

FOOD DESCRIPTION	MEASURE OR QUANTITY	FATS IN GRAMS		
		Total	Saturated	Unsaturated
DANDELION GREENS, raw (USDA):				
Trimmed	1 lb.	3.2		
Boiled, drained	½ cup (3.2 oz.)	.5		
DANISH PASTRY (See **CAKE,** Coffee, or **ROLL & BUN**)				
DATE, dry:				
Domestic:				
With pits (USDA)	1 lb. (weighed with pits)	2.0		
Without pits (USDA)	4 oz.	.6		
Whole (Cal-Date)	4 oz.	.7		
Imported, Iraq (Bordo):				
Whole	4 average dates (.9 oz.)	.6		
Diced	¼ cup (2 oz.)	1.4		
DELAWARE WINE	Any quantity	0.0		
DENNY'S:				
BLT	1 serving	33.0		
Chef salad	1 serving	22.0		
Chicken:				
Sandwich, breast	1 serving	47.0		
Steak, fried	1 serving	62.0		
Stir fry	1 serving	43.0		
Club sandwich	1 serving	35.0		
Denny Burger	1 serving	44.0		
Egg, omelet, made with *Egg Beaters*	1 serving	59.0		
Grand Slam	1 serving	59.0		
Halibut	1 serving	28.0		
Patty melt	1 serving	45.0		
Super Bird	1 serving	29.0		
Turkey sandwich, sliced	1 serving	26.0		
DEWBERRY PRESERVE (Bama)	1 T. (.7 oz.)	Tr.		
DINERSAURS, cereal (Ralston-Purina)	1 cup (1 oz.)	1		
DINNER, frozen (See individual listings such as **BEEF DINNER, CHICKEN DINNER, CHINESE DINNER, ENCHILADA DINNER,** etc.)				
DIP:				
Acapulco (Ortega):				
Plain	1 oz.	.1		
American cheese	1 oz.	4.6		
Bean (Eagle)	1 oz.	2.0		
Blue cheese (Breakstone's)	1 oz.	5.2		
Chili (La Victoria)	1 T.	Tr.		
Chili bean (Old El Paso)	1 T.	Tr.		
Guacamole (Calavo)	1 oz.	4.0		
Hot bean (Hain)	1 T.	Tr.		
Jalapeño:				
Fritos	1 oz.	1.7		
(Wise)	1 T.	0.0		
Onion (Thank You Brand)	1 T.	3.6		
Onion bean (Hain)	1 oz.	2.0		
Picante sauce (Wise)	1 T.	0.0		
Taco:				
(Old El Paso)	1 T.	Tr.		
(Wise)	1 T.	0.0		
DOUGHNUT:				
(USDA):				
Cake type	1.1-oz piece	6.0	0.0	5.0
Yeast leavened	2 oz.	15.1	3.0	12.0
(Dolly Madison):				
Regular:				
Plain	1¼-oz. piece	7.0		
Chocolate-coated	1¼-oz. piece	8.0		
Coconut crunch	1¼-oz. piece	5.0		
Powdered sugar	1¼-oz. piece	6.0		
Dunkin' Stix	1⅜-oz. piece	15.0		

FOOD DESCRIPTION	MEASURE OR QUANTITY	FATS IN GRAMS		
		Total	Saturated	Unsaturated
Gems:				
Chocolate-coated	.5-oz. piece	4.0		
Cinnamon sugar or coconut crunch	.5-oz. piece	2.5		
Powdered sugar	.5-oz. piece	3.0		
Jumbo:				
Plain or sugar	1.6-oz. piece	10.0		
Cinnamon sugar	1.6-oz. piece	9.0		
Old-fashioned:				
Cinnamon chip, glazed or crush	2.2-oz. piece	15.0		
Chocolate-glazed	2.2-oz. piece	12.0		
Powdered sugar or white iced	1 piece	17.0		
DUCK, raw (USDA):				
Domesticated:				
Meat & skin	4 oz.	32.4		
Meat only	4 oz.	9.3		
Wild:				
Dressed	1 lb. (weighed dressed)	41.6		
Meat, skin & giblets	4 oz.	17.9		
Meat only	4 oz.	5.9		
ECLAIR, home recipe, with custard filling & chocolate icing (USDA)	4 oz.	15.4	5.0	11.0
EEL (USDA):				
Raw, meat only	4 oz.	20.8	5.0	16.0
Smoked, meat only	4 oz.	31.5	7.0	25.0
EGG, CHICKEN (USDA):				
Raw:				
White only	1 large egg (1.2 oz.)	Tr.		
Yolk only	1 large egg (.6 oz.)	5.2	2.0	4.0
Yolk only	1 cup (8.5 oz.)	73.4	24.0	49.0
Whole, small	1 egg (1.3 oz.)	4.3	1.0	3.0
Whole, large	1 egg (1.8 oz.)	5.7	2.0	4.0
Whole, extra large	1 egg (2 oz.)	6.6	2.0	4.0
Whole, jumbo	1 egg (2.3 oz.)	7.4	3.0	5.0
Cooked:				
Boiled	1 large egg (1.8 oz.)	5.7	2.0	4.0
Fried in butter	1 large egg (1.6 oz.)	7.9	3.0	5.0
Omelet, mixed with milk & cooked in fat	1 large egg (2.2 oz.)	8.0	3.0	5.0
Poached	1 large egg (1.7 oz.)	5.6	2.0	4.0
Scrambled, mixed with milk & cooked in fat	1 cup (7.8 oz.)	28.4	11.0	17.0
Scrambled, mixed with milk & cooked in fat	1 large egg (2.3 oz.)	8.3	3.0	5.0
Dried:				
White, flakes or powder	1 oz.	Tr.		
Yolk	1 cup (3.4 oz.)	54.3	17.0	37.0
Whole	1 cup (3.8 oz.)	44.5	14.0	30.0
Whole, glucose reduced	1 oz.	12.2	4.0	8.0
Frozen, whole, raw	1 oz.	3.3	1.0	2.0
EGG, DUCK, raw (USDA)	1 egg (2.8 oz.)	11.6		
EGG, GOOSE, raw (USDA)	1 egg (5.8 oz.)	21.8		
EGG, TURKEY, raw (USDA)	1 egg (3.1 oz.)	10.4		
EGG, BREAKFAST OR ENTREE, frozen (Swanson):				
Omelet:				
With cheese & ham	7-oz. meal	31.0		
Spanish style	7¾-oz. meal	17.0		
Scrambled, with sausage & hash-brown potatoes	6¼-oz. meal	33.0		
*EGG FOO YOUNG, canned:				
(Chun King) stir fry	5-oz. serving	8.2		
(La Choy)	1 patty & ¼ cup sauce	7.0		
EGG NOG, dairy (Borden's)	½ cup (4.2 oz.)	9.0		
EGG NOG COCKTAIL (Mr. Boston) 15% alcohol	3 fl. oz.	2.1		

FOOD DESCRIPTION	MEASURE OR QUANTITY	FATS IN GRAMS		
		Total	Saturated	Unsaturated
EGGPLANT:				
Boiled, drained (USDA)	4 oz.	.2		
Boiled, drained, diced (USDA)	1 cup (7.1 oz.)	.4		
Frozen:				
(Buitoni) parmigiana	5-oz. serving	8.7		
(Celentano):				
Parmigiana	½ of 16-oz. pkg.	15.0		
Rollettes	11-oz. pkg.	14.0		
EGG ROLL, frozen:				
(Chun King):				
Regular:				
Chicken or meat & shrimp	3½-oz. piece	8.0		
Shrimp	3½-oz. piece	6.0		
Restaurant-style, pork	3-oz. piece	6.0		
(La Choy):				
Chicken	.5-oz. piece	1.0		
Lobster	3-oz. piece	5.0		
Shrimp	3-oz. piece	4.0		
EGG SUBSTITUTE:				
Egg Beaters (Fleischmann's):				
Cholesterol-free	¼ cup	0.0		
With cheese, 99% real egg product	½ cup	6.0		
Scramblers (Morningstar Farms)	1 egg equivalent	1.5		
ELDERBERRY, fresh (USDA) stems removed	4 oz.	.6		
EL POLLO LOCO, restaurant:				
Beans	3½-oz. serving	1.0	1.0	
Chicken, 2-piece	4.8-oz. serving (edible portion)	18.0		
Combo	16-oz. serving (edible portion)	28.0		
Corn	3.3-oz. serving	2.0		
Dole whip	4½-oz. serving	0.0		
Potato salad	4.3-oz. serving	8.0		
Rice	2½-oz. serving	1.0		
Salsa	1.8-oz. serving	0.0		
Tortilla:				
Corn	3.3-oz. serving	2.0		
Flour	3.3-oz. serving	7.0		
ENCHILADA OR ENCHILADA DINNER:				
Canned (Old El Paso) beef, with filling	1 enchilada	8.0	3.0	1.0
Frozen:				
Bean & beef (Stouffer's) *Lean Cuisine*	9¼-oz. meal	10.0		
Beef:				
(Banquet) dinner	12-oz. meal	15.0		
Marquez (Fred's Frozen Foods)	7½-oz. serving	13.3		
(Old El Paso) dinner	11-oz. dinner	8.0		
(Patio)	13¼-oz. meal	24.0		
(Weight Watchers)	9.1-oz. meal	13.0	4.0	9.0
Cheese:				
(Old El Paso) dinner	11-oz. dinner	31.0		
(Patio)	12¼-oz. dinner	10.0		
(Weight Watchers)	8.87-oz. meal	18.0	5.0	13.0
Chicken:				
(Old El Paso):				
Dinner	11-oz. dinner	18.0		
Entree, with sour cream sauce	1 piece	19.0		
(Weight Watchers) Suiza	9.37-oz. meal	15.0	6.0	9.0
ENCHILADA SAUCE, canned:				
(El Molino) hot	1 T.	.5		
(La Victoria)	1 T.	Tr.		

FOOD DESCRIPTION	MEASURE OR QUANTITY	FATS IN GRAMS		
		Total	Saturated	Unsaturated
ENCHILADA SEASONING MIX				
(Lawry's)	1.6-oz. pkg.	1.2		
ENDIVE, CURLY, OR ESCAROLE, raw (USDA):				
Untrimmed	1 lb. (weighed untrimmed)	.4		
Cut up or shredded	1 cup (2.5 oz.)	Tr.		
ESCAROLE (See **ENDIVE**)				
FAJITA, frozen:				
(Healthy Choice):				
Beef	7-oz. serving	4.0	2.0	Tr.
Chicken	7-oz. serving	3.0	1.0	1.0
(Weight Watchers):				
Beef	6¾-oz. serving	7.0	2.0	5.0
Chicken	6¾-oz. serving	5.0	2.0	3.0
FAJITA SEASONING MIX				
(Lawry's)	1.3-oz. pkg.	.4		
FARINA (See also **CREAM OF WHEAT**):				
Regular:				
Dry:				
(USDA)	1 cup (6 oz.)	1.5		
(H-O) cream, enriched	1 cup (6.1 oz.)	Tr.		
Cooked:				
(USDA)	1 cup (8.4 oz.)	.2		
(Pillsbury)	⅔ cup (1 oz. dry)	.2		
Quick-cooking (USDA) cooked	1 cup (8.5 oz.)	.2		
Instant-cooking (USDA) cooked	4 oz.	.1		
FAT, COOKING:				
(USDA):				
Lard	1 lb.	454.0	172.0	282.0
Lard	1 cup (7.2 oz.)	205.0	78.0	127.0
Vegetable	1 cup (7.1 oz.)	200.0	50.0	150.0
Vegetable	1 T. (.4 oz.)	12.0	3.0	9.0
Crisco	2 T. (.4 oz.)	11.7	3.0	9.0
Light Spray	1 T. (.4 oz.)	10.6	3.0	8.0
FENNEL LEAVES, raw (USDA) trimmed	4 oz.	.5		
FETTUCINI, frozen:				
(Armour Classics) *Dining Lite,* & broccoli	9-oz. pkg.	12.0		
(Green Giant) primavera	9½-oz. pkg.	8.0	3.0	3.0
(Healthy Choice) alfredo	8-oz. pkg.	6.0	2.0	3.0
(Stouffer's) alfredo	½ of 10-oz. pkg.	19.0		
FIBER ONE, cereal (General Mills)	½ cup (1 oz.)	1.0		
FIG:				
Fresh (USDA)	1.3-oz. fig (1½")	.1		
Candied (USDA)	1 oz.	Tr.		
Canned, regular pack, solids & liq.:				
(USDA)	½ cup (4.4 oz.)	.3		
(Stokely-Van Camp's)	½ cup (4.2 oz.)	.2		
Dried:				
(USDA):				
Whole	.7-oz. fig (2" × 1")	.3		
Chopped	1 cup (6 oz.)	2.2		
(Sun-Maid) Calimyrna	½ cup	2.0		
FILBERT OR HAZELNUT				
(USDA) shelled	1 oz.	17.7	Tr.	17.0
FINNAN HADDIE (See **HADDOCK, SMOKED**)				
FISH (See individual listings)				
'FISH BOUILLON (Knorr's)	8 fl. oz.	.4		
FISH CAKE:				
Home recipe (USDA) fried	2 oz.	4.5		
Frozen:				
(USDA) fried, reheated	2 oz.	10.1		
(Mrs. Paul's) regular	1 cake	4.0		

FOOD DESCRIPTION	MEASURE OR QUANTITY	FATS IN GRAMS		
		Total	Saturated	Unsaturated
FISH & CHIPS, frozen:				
(Gorton's)	1 pkg.	72.0		
(Mrs. Paul's)	14-oz. pkg.	21.4		
FISH DINNER OR ENTREE, frozen:				
(Banquet) platter	8¾-oz. meal	22.0		
(Gorton's):				
Fillet almondine	1 pkg.	25.0	10.0	15.0
Fillet, in herb butter	1 pkg.	8.0	5.0	2.0
(Kid Cuisine) nuggets	7-oz. pkg.	15.0		
(Stouffer's) *Lean Cuisine:*				
Divan	12⅜-oz. pkg.	7.0		
Florentine	9-oz. pkg.	9.0		
(Weight Watchers):				
Au gratin	9¼-oz. meal	6.0	1.0	5.0
Oven fried	7.1-oz. serving	13.0	Tr.	13.0
FISH FILLET, frozen:				
(Gorton's):				
Regular:				
Batter dipped, crispy	1 piece	10.0	4.0	7.0
Microwave	1 piece	13.0	6.0	7.0
Light Recipe:				
Lightly breaded	1 piece	8.0	3.0	5.0
Tempura batter	1 piece	14.0	4.0	10.0
(Van de Kamp's):				
Batter dipped, french fried	3-oz. piece	10.0		
Light & crunchy	2-oz. piece	15.0		
FISH FLAKES, canned (USDA)	4 oz.	.7		
FISH KABOB, frozen (Van de Kamp's)	1 piece	15.0		
FISH LOAF, home recipe (USDA)	4 oz.	4.2		
FISH STICK, frozen:				
(Gorton's) potato crisp	1 piece	4.0	1.2	2.7
(Van de Kamp's) batter dipped, Light & Crispy	1 piece	5.0		
FLOUNDER:				
Raw (USDA) meat only	4 oz.	.9		
Baked (USDA)	4 oz.	9.3		
Frozen:				
(Gorton's):				
Fishmarket Fresh	4 oz.	1.0		
Microwave entree, stuffed	1 pkg.	18.0	7.0	11.0
(Van de Kamp's) *Today's Catch*	4 oz.	0.0		
FLOUR:				
(USDA):				
Buckwheat, dark, sifted	1 cup (3.5 oz.)	2.4		
Buckwheat, light, sifted	1 cup (3.5 oz.)	1.2		
Carob or St. John's-bread	1 oz.	.4		
Chestnut	1 oz.	1.0		
Corn, sifted	1 cup (3.9 oz.)	2.9	Tr.	3.0
Cottonseed	1 oz.	1.9	Tr.	1.0
Rye:				
Light:				
Unsifted, spooned	1 cup (3.6 oz.)	1.0		
Sifted, spooned	1 cup (3.1 oz.)	.9		
Medium	1 oz.	.5		
Dark, stirred or unstirred	1 cup (4.5 oz.)	3.3		
Soybean:				
Defatted, stirred	1 cup (3.6 oz.)	.9		
Low-fat, stirred	1 cup (3.1 oz.)	5.9	Tr.	5.0
Full fat, stirred	1 cup (2.5 oz.)	14.6	2.0	12.0
Sunflower seed, partially defatted	1 oz.	1.0	Tr.	1.0
Tapioca, unsifted, spooned	1 cup (3.8 oz.)	.2		
Wheat:				
All-purpose	1 oz.	.3		
Sifted, spooned	1 cup (4.1 oz.)	1.1		

FOOD DESCRIPTION	MEASURE OR QUANTITY	FATS IN GRAMS		
		Total	Saturated	Unsaturated
Bread:				
Unsifted, dipped	1 cup (4.8 oz.)	1.5		
Sifted, spooned	1 cup (4.1 oz.)	1.3		
Cake or pastry:				
Unsifted, dipped	1 cup (4.2 oz.)	1.0		
Sifted, spooned	1 cup (3.5 oz.)	.8		
Gluton:				
Unsifted, dipped	1 cup (5 oz.)	2.7		
Sifted, spooned	1 cup (3.8 oz.)	2.6		
Self-rising, unsifted, dipped	1 cup (4.6 oz.)	1.3		
Whole wheat, stirred, spooned	1 cup (4.8 oz.)	2.7		
Aunt Jemima, self-rising	1 cup (4 oz.)	1.2		
Gold Medal (Betty Crocker):				
Regular, better for bread or self-rising	1 cup	1.4		
Wondra	1 cup	1.4		
Presto, self-rising	1 cup (3.9 oz.)	.9		
(Quaker)	1 cup (4 oz.)	1.2		
FRANKENBERRY, cereal (General Mills)	1 cup (1 oz.)	1.0		
FRANKFURTER OR WIENER:				
(Eckrich):				
Beef	1.6-oz. frankfurter	13.0		
Meat	1.2-oz. frankfurter	11.0		
Hebrew National:				
Beef:				
Regular	1.7-oz. frankfurter	14.0		
Light	1.7-oz. frankfurter	10.0		
Collagen	2.3-oz. frankfurter	19.0		
(Hygrade) beef, *Ball Park*	2-oz. frankfurter	15.6		
(Louis Rich) turkey	1.5-oz. frankfurter	8.0		
(Oscar Mayer):				
Beef	1.6-oz. frankfurter	13.2	5.6	7.3
& cheese	1.6-oz. frankfurter	11.3	5.1	5.9
Little Wiener	2″ frankfurter	2.6		
FRANKS & BEANS (See **BEANS & FRANKS**)				
FRENCH TOAST, frozen:				
(Aunt Jemima) regular	1 slice (1.5 oz.)	2.2		
(Swanson) plain	6½-oz. breakfast	26.0		
FRITTERS:				
Apple, frozen (Mrs. Paul's)	2-oz. fritter	7.5		
Clam, home recipe (USDA)	1.4-oz. fritter	6.0		
Corn, home recipe (USDA)	1 fritter (1.2 oz.)	24.4	5.7	18.7
FROG LEGS, raw (USDA):				
Bone in	1 lb. (weighed with bone)	.9		
Meat only	4 oz.	.3		
FROOT LOOPS, cereal (Kellogg's)	1 cup (1 oz.)	1.0		
FROSTING (See **CAKE ICING**)				
FROZEN CUSTARD (See **ICE CREAM**)				
FROZEN DESSERT (See also *TOFUTTI*):				
(Baskin-Robbins) *Low, Lite'n Luscious,* chunky banana	½ cup	1.0		
(Borden's) ice milk, strawberry or vanilla	½ cup	2.0		
Mocha Mix (Presto Food Products):				
Bar, vanilla, chocolate-covered	4-fl.-oz. bar	16.0	3.0	13.0
Bulk:				
Berry, peach or strawberry swirl	4 fl. oz.	6.0	1.0	5.0
Dutch chocolate or mocha almond fudge	4 fl. oz.	8.0	2.0	6.0
Neapolitan or vanilla	4 fl. oz.	7.0	2.0	5.0

FOOD DESCRIPTION	MEASURE OR QUANTITY	FATS IN GRAMS		
		Total	Saturated	Unsaturated
FRUIT COCKTAIL, canned, regular pack, solids & liq.:				
(USDA) light, heavy, extra heavy syrup or water pack	½ cup	.1		
(Del Monte) heavy syrup	½ cup	.1		
FRUIT COMPOTE (Rokeach)	½ cup (4 oz.)	1.0		
FRUIT & CREAM BAR (Dole):				
Blueberry, peach, raspberry or strawberry	1 bar	1.0		
Chocolate-banana	1 bar	9.0		
Chocolate-strawberry	1 bar	8.0		
FRUIT & FIBRE, cereal (Post):				
Dates, raisins, walnuts with oat clusters or whole wheat & bran flakes with peaches, raisins, almonds & oat clusters	⅔ cup (1¼ oz.)	2.0		
Tropical fruit with oat clusters	⅔ cup (1¼ oz.)	3.0		
FRUIT & JUICE BAR, frozen:				
(Dole) *Fresh Lites, Fruit 'n Juice* or *Sun Tops*	1 bar	Tr		
(Weight Watchers)	1.7-fl.-oz. bar	0.0		
FRUIT, MIXED:				
Canned:				
(Hunt's) *Snack-Pak*	5-oz. container	Tr.		
(Libby's) lite	½ cup	1.0		
Dried:				
(Del Monte)	2 oz.	0.0		
(Sun-Maid/Sunsweet)	2 oz.	Tr.		
FRUIT PUNCH:				
Canned (Hi-C)	6 fl. oz.	Tr.		
*Mix, dietetic *Crystal Light*	6 fl. oz.	Tr.		
FRUIT ROLL (Flavor Tree)	¾-oz. piece	Tr.		
FRUIT SALAD:				
Bottled, chilled (Kraft)	4 oz.	.1		
Canned, regular pack, solids & liq.:				
(USDA) light, heavy or extra heavy syrup	½ cup	.1		
(Del Monte)	½ cup	0.0		
FRUIT SLUSH (Wyler's) any flavor	4 fl. oz.	0.0		
FRUITYYUMMYMUMMY, cereal (General Mills)	1 cup (1 oz.)	1.0		
GARBANZO, dry (See **CHICK PEA,** dry)				
GARFIELD AND FRIENDS (General Mills):				
Pouch:				
1–2 Punch	.9-oz. pouch	2.0		
Very strawberry	.9-oz. pouch	1.0		
Roll	.5-oz. roll	Tr.		
GARLIC, raw (USDA) peeled	1 oz.	Tr.		
GARLIC POWDER (Lawry's)	1 tsp.	Tr.		
GARLIC SPREAD (Lawry's):				
Concentrate	1 T.	1.6		
Ready-to-use, bread spread	1 T.	9.2		
GEFILTE FISH:				
(Mother's) any type	4 oz.	1.0		
(Rokeach):				
Natural broth	2-oz. piece	.8		
Jelled	1 piece	.6		
GELATIN, unflavored, dry (Knox)	7-gram envelope	0.0		
GELATIN DESSERT MIX:				
*(Jell-O) any flavor	½ cup	Tr.		
*(Royal) any flavor	½ cup	0.0		
GELATIN DRINK, plain or flavored (Knox)	1 envelope (.7 oz.)	0.0		

FOOD DESCRIPTION	MEASURE OR QUANTITY	FATS IN GRAMS		
		Total	Saturated	Unsaturated
GINGERBREAD, home recipe (USDA):				
Made with butter	1.9-oz. piece (2″ × 2″ × 2″)	5.3	3.0	3.0
Made with vegetable shortening	1.9-oz. piece (2″ × 2″ × 2″)	5.9	2.0	4.0
GINGERBREAD MIX:				
*(Betty Crocker) regular or no-cholesterol recipe	⅑ of cake	7.0	2.0	<5.0
*(Dromedary)	1.2-oz. piece (2″ × 2″)	2.0		
GINGER ROOT, fresh (USDA) with or without skin	1 oz.	.3		
GOOSE, domesticated (USDA):				
Roasted, meat & skin	4 oz.	43.2		
Roasted, meat only	4 oz.	11.1		
GOOSE, GIBLET, raw (USDA)	4 oz.	7.9		
GOOSE GIZZARD, raw (USDA)	4 oz.	6.0		
GRANOLA BAR:				
Nature Valley:				
Cinnamon or oats'n honey	1 bar	5.0		
Oat bran-honey graham	1 bar	4.0		
New Trail (Hershey's) chocolate covered:				
Chocolate chip or cookies & cream	1.2-oz. piece	8.0		
Peanut butter	1.3-oz. piece	10.0		
GRANOLA CEREAL:				
Nature Valley, cinnamon & raisin, fruit & nut or toasted oats	⅓ cup (1 oz.)	5.0		
Sun Country (Kretschmer):				
With almonds	¼ cup (1 oz.)	4.8		
With raisins	¼ cup (1 oz.)	4.5		
GRANOLA SNACK, *Kudos* (M&M/Mars):				
Chocolate chip	1¼-oz. serving	9.0		
Peanut butter	1.3-oz. serving	12.0		
GRAPE:				
Fresh (USDA):				
American type (slip skin), Concord, Delaware, Niagara, Catawba & Scuppernong, pulp only	½ lb. (weighed with stem, skin & seeds)	1.4		
European type (adherent skin) Malaga, Muscat, Thompson seedless, Emperor & Flame Tokay, with skin	½ lb. (weighed with stems & seeds)	.6		
Canned, solids & liq. (USDA) Thompson seedless, heavy syrup or water pack	4 oz.	.1		
GRAPEADE (Minute Maid) chilled or frozen	6 fl. oz.	Tr.		
GRAPEFRUIT:				
Fresh, pulp only (USDA):				
Seeded or seedless	1 lb. (weighed with seeds and skin)	.2		
Seeded or seedless	½ med. grapefruit (3¾″, 8.5 oz.)	.1		
Bottled, chilled, sections (Kraft) sweetened or unsweetened	4 oz.	.1		
Canned, sections, syrup pack, solids & liq.:				
(USDA)	½ cup (4.5 oz.)	.1		
(Stokely-Van Camp's) light syrup	½ cup (4 oz.)	.1		

FOOD DESCRIPTION	MEASURE OR QUANTITY	FATS IN GRAMS		
		Total	Saturated	Unsaturated
GRAPEFRUIT JUICE:				
Fresh (USDA) pink, red or white, all varieties	½ cup (4.3 oz.)	.1		
Bottled, chilled (Kraft) sweetened or unsweetened	½ cup (4.3 oz.)	.1		
Canned:				
(USDA)	½ cup (4.4 oz.)	.1		
(Del Monte)	½ cup	Tr.		
*Frozen (Minute Maid)	½ cup (4.2 oz.)	Tr.		
GRAPEFRUIT-ORANGE JUICE (See ORANGE-GRAPEFRUIT JUICE)				
GRAPEFRUIT PEEL, CANDIED (USDA)	1 oz.	Tr.		
GRAPE JAM, sweetened (Smucker's)	1 T. (.7 oz.)	Tr.		
GRAPE JELLY, low-calorie (Kraft)	1 oz.	Tr.		
GRAPE JUICE:				
Canned (Heinz)	5½-fl.-oz. can	.2		
*Frozen (Snow Crop)	½ cup (4.2 oz.)	Tr.		
GRAPE-NUTS, cereal (Post):				
Regular or raisin	¼ cup (1 oz.)	Tr.		
Flakes	⅞ cup (1 oz.)	.9	.4	.2
GRAVY, canned:				
Au jus (Franco-American)	2 oz.	0.0		
Beef (Franco-American)	2 oz.	1.0		
Brown (Estee) dietetic	¼ cup	0.0		
Chicken (Franco-American) regular	2 oz.	4.0		
Turkey (Franco-American)	2 oz.	2.0		
GRAVY MASTER	1 fl. oz.	Tr.		
GRAVY WITH MEAT OR TURKEY, frozen (Banquet):				
Cookin' Bags:				
& salisbury steak	5-oz. pkg.	14.0		
& sliced beef	4-oz. pkg.	5.0		
& sliced turkey	5-oz. pkg.	6.0		
Family Entree:				
Onion gravy & beef patties	¼ of 32-oz. pkg.	21.0		
& sliced beef	¼ of 32-oz. pkg.	5.0		
& sliced turkey	¼ of 32-oz. pkg.	8.0		
*GRAVY MIX:				
Au jus (Durkee)	1 cup	.1		
Brown:				
(Knorr) classic	3 fl. oz.	.9		
(Lawry's)	½ cup	.7		
Chicken:				
(Durkee)	1 cup	2.3		
(French's)	¼ cup	1.2		
Homestyle (French's)	¼ cup	1.0		
Turkey (French's)	¼ cup	1.0		
GREENS, MIXED, canned, solids & liq. (Allen)	½ cup (4 oz.)	Tr.		
GRITS (See HOMINY GRITS)				
GROUPER, raw (USDA) meat only	4 oz.	.6		
GUACAMOLE SEASONING MIX (Lawry's)	.7-oz. pkg.	.4		
GUAVA, COMMON, fresh (USDA) flesh only	4 oz.	.7		
GUAVA FRUIT DRINK, canned, *Mauna La'I*	6 fl. oz.	0.0		
GUAVA NECTAR, canned (Libby's)	6 fl. oz.	0.0		
GUINEA HEN, raw (USDA):				
Meat & skin	4 oz.	7.3		
Giblets	2 oz.	4.0		
GUM (See CHEWING GUM)				

FOOD DESCRIPTION	MEASURE OR QUANTITY	FATS IN GRAMS		
		Total	Saturated	Unsaturated
HADDOCK:				
Raw (USDA) meat only	4 oz.	.1		
Fried, dipped in egg, milk & bread crumbs (USDA)	4" × 3" × 1/2" fillet (3.5 oz.)	6.4		
Frozen:				
(Gorton's):				
Fishmarket Fresh	4 oz.	1.0		
Microwave entree in lemon butter	1 pkg.	21.0	10.0	11.0
(Van de Kamp's) batter dipped	2 oz.	5.0		
Smoked, canned or not, (USDA)	4 oz.	.5		
HALIBUT (USDA):				
Raw, Atlantic & Pacific:				
Whole	1 lb. (weighed whole)	3.2		
Meat only, not dipped or dipped in brine	4 oz.	1.4		
Broiled with vegetable shortening	6½" × 2½" × 8" or 4" × 3" × 1/2" steak (4.4 oz.)	8.8		
Smoked	4 oz.	17.0		
HAM (See also **PORK**):				
Boiled:				
Luncheon Meat (USDA)[1]	1 oz.	4.8	2.0	3.0
Luncheon meat, chopped (USDA)[1]	1 cup (4.8 oz.)	23.1	8.0	15.0
Luncheon meat, diced (USDA)[1]	1 cup (5 oz.)	24.0	8.0	16.0
(Hormel)	1 oz.	1.4	Tr.	<1.0
Chopped, sliced (Hormel)	1 oz.	5.8		
Minced (Oscar Mayer)	1 slice (10 per 1/2 lb.)	4.4		
Smoked (Oscar Mayer)	1 slice (8 per 6 oz.)	1.5		
Smoked, thin sliced (Oscar Mayer)	1 slice (10 per 3 oz.)	.6		
Canned:				
(USDA)	1 oz.	3.5	1.0	2.0
(Armour Star)	1 oz.	3.5		
(Hormel)	1 oz. (6-lb. can)	2.6		
(Hormel)	1 oz. (1-lb. 8-oz. can)	3.1		
(Oscar Mayer) *Jubilee*, bone in	1 lb.	54.4		
(Oscar Mayer) *Jubilee*, special trim, as purchased	1 oz.	2.3		
(Oscar Mayer) *Jubilee*, special trim, cooked	1 oz.	1.4	<1.0	<1.0
(Oscar Mayer) steak	1 slice (8 to lb.)	3.4		
(Swift)	1¾-oz. slice (5" × 2¼" × 1/4")	7.8		
(Swift) *Hostess*	1 oz. (4-lb. can)	1.6		
Chopped or minced, canned:				
(USDA)[1]	1 oz.	4.8	2.0	3.0
(Hormel)	1 oz. (8-lb. can)	7.9	3.0	5.0
(Oscar Mayer)	1-oz. slice	4.8		
Chopped, spiced or unspiced, canned:				
(USDA)[1]	1 oz.	7.1	3.0	5.0
Chopped (USDA)[1]	1 cup (4.8 oz.)	33.9	12.0	22.0
Diced (USDA)[1]	1 cup (5 oz.)	35.1	13.0	22.0
(Hormel)	1 oz. (5-lb. can)	6.6		
Deviled, canned:				
(USDA)[1]	1 oz.	9.2	3.0	6.0
(USDA)[1]	1 T. (.5 oz.)	4.2	2.0	3.0
(Hormel)	1 oz. (3-oz. can)	6.1		
(Underwood)	1 T. (.5 oz.)	4.3		

[1]Principal source of fat: pork.

FOOD DESCRIPTION	MEASURE OR QUANTITY	FATS IN GRAMS		
		Total	Saturated	Unsaturated
Packaged:				
(Carl Buddig) smoked, sliced	1 oz.	3.0	.8	2.0
(Eckrich):				
Chopped:				
Regular	1-oz. slice	2.0		
Smorgas Pak	3/4-oz. slice	2.0		
Cooked	1.2-oz. slice	1.0		
Loaf	1-oz. slice	6.0		
Smoked, sweet:				
Regular	3/4-oz. slice	1.0		
Slender-sliced	1-oz. serving	3.0		
(Hormel):				
Black-peppered, *Light & Lean*	1 slice	1.0		
Cooked, *Light & Lean*	1 slice	1.0		
Red peppered, *Light & Lean*	1 slice	1.0		
(Ohse):				
Chopped	1 oz.	5.0		
Smoked:				
Regular	1 oz.	3.0		
95% fat free	1 oz.	1.0		
Turkey ham	1 oz.	1.0		
(Oscar Mayer):				
Chopped	1-oz. slice	4.5		
Smoked, cooked	3/4-oz. slice	1.1		
Steak, boneless, 95% fat-free *Jubilee*	2-oz. serving	2.2		
HAM & CHEESE:				
Canned (Hormel) loaf	3 oz.	22.0		
Packaged:				
(Eckrich) loaf	1-oz. slice	5.0		
(Oscar Mayer) loaf	1-oz. slice	6.2		
HAM CROQUETTE, home recipe (USDA)	4 oz.	17.1	7.0	10.0
HAM DINNER, frozen:				
(Armour) *Dinner Classics,* steak	10 3/4-oz. pkg.	7.0		
(Morton)	10-oz. pkg.	34.0		
HAM SPREAD, salad:				
(Carnation) *Spreadables*	1/4 of 7 1/2-oz. can	8.0		
(Oscar Mayer)	1 oz.	3.8	1.3	2.6
*HAMBURGER SEASONING MIX,				
Hamburger Helper:				
Beef noodle, hamburger hash, potato stroganoff, *Sloppy Joe Bake,* spaghetti or *Tacobake*	1/5 of pkg.	15.0		
Beef romanoff or tamale pie	1/5 of pkg.	16.0		
Chili tomato, hamburger pizza dish or stew	1/5 of pkg.	14.0		
Italian:				
Cheesy	1/5 of pkg.	17.0		
Zesty	1/5 of pkg.	13.0		
Meat loaf	1/5 of pkg.	22.0		
HARDEE'S:				
Apple turnover	3.2-oz. piece	12.0	4.0	8.0
Big Cookie	1.7-oz. serving	13.0	4.0	9.0
Big Country Breakfast:				
Bacon	7.6-oz. serving	40.0	10.0	30.0
Country ham	9-oz. serving	38.0	9.0	29.0
Ham	8.8-oz. serving	33.0	7.0	27.0
Sausage	9.7-oz. serving	57.0	16.0	42.0
Big Twin	6.1-oz. serving	25.0	11.0	14.0
Biscuit:				
Bacon	3.3-oz. serving	21.0	4.0	17.0
Bacon & egg	4.4-oz. serving	24.0	5.0	19.0
Bacon, egg & cheese	4.8-oz. serving	28.0	8.0	20.0
Chicken	5.1-oz. serving	22.0	4.0	18.0

FOOD DESCRIPTION	MEASURE OR QUANTITY	FATS IN GRAMS		
		Total	Saturated	Unsaturated
Cinnamon 'N' Raisin	2.8-oz. serving	17.0	5.0	12.0
Country ham	3.8-oz. serving	18.0	3.0	15.0
Country ham & egg	4.9-oz. serving	22.0	4.0	17.0
Ham	3.7-oz. serving	16.0	2.0	14.0
Ham & egg	4.9-oz. serving	19.0	4.0	16.0
Ham, egg & cheese	1 serving	23.0	6.0	17.0
Rise 'N' Shine:				
Regular	2.9-oz. serving	18.0	3.0	15.0
Canadian	5.7-oz. serving	27.0	8.0	20.0
Sausage	4.2-oz. serving	28.0	7.0	21.0
Sausage & egg	5.3-oz. serving	31.0	8.0	24.0
Steak	5.2-oz. serving	29.0	7.0	22.0
Steak & egg	5.1-oz. serving	22.0	4.0	18.0
Biscuit 'N' Gravy	7.8-oz. serving	24.0	6.0	19.0
Cheeseburger:				
Plain	4.3-oz. serving	14.0	7.0	7.0
Bacon	7.7-oz. serving	39.0	16.0	23.0
Quarter-pound	6.4-oz. serving	29.0	14.0	14.0
Chicken fillet	6.1-oz. serving	13.0	2.0	10.0
Chicken sandwich, grilled	6.8-oz. serving	9.0	1.0	8.0
Chicken Stix:				
6-piece	3½-oz. serving	9.0	2.0	7.0
9-piece	5.3-oz. serving	14.0	3.0	11.0
Cool Twist:				
Cone, any flavor	4.2-oz. serving	6.0	4.0	2.0
Sundae:				
Caramel	5.9-oz. serving	10.0	5.0	4.0
Hot fudge	5.9-oz. serving	12.0	6.0	5.0
Strawberry	5.8-oz. serving	8.0	5.0	4.0
Fisherman's Fillet	7.3-oz. serving	24.0	6.0	18.0
Hamburger:				
Regular	3.9-oz. serving	10.0	4.0	6.0
Big deluxe	7.6-oz. serving	30.0	12.0	17.0
Mushroom & swiss	6.7-oz. serving	27.0	13.0	14.0
Ham & cheese, hot	5¼-oz. serving	12.0	5.0	6.0
Hot dog, all beef	4.2-oz. serving	17.0	8.0	10.0
Margarine/butter blend	5-gram serving	4.0	Tr.	2.0
Pancakes, three:				
Plain	4.8-oz. serving	2.0	1.0	1.0
With 2 bacon strips	5.3-oz. serving	9.0	3.0	5.0
With 1 sausage patty	6.2-oz. serving	16.0	6.0	10.0
Potato:				
Big Fry	5½-oz. serving	23.0	5.0	19.0
Crispy Curls	3-oz. serving	16.0	3.0	13.0
French fries:				
Regular order	2½-oz. serving	11.0	2.0	9.0
Large	4-oz. serving	17.0	3.0	13.0
Hash Rounds	2.8-oz. serving	14.0	3.0	11.0
Roast beef:				
Regular	4-oz. serving	9.0	4.0	6.0
Big	4.7-oz. serving	11.0	5.0	7.0
Salad:				
Chef	10.4-oz. serving	15.0	9.0	6.0
Chicken & pasta	14.6-oz. serving	3.0	1.0	2.0
Garden	8½-oz. serving	14.0	8.0	6.0
Side	4-oz. serving	Tr.	Tr.	Tr.
Shake:				
Chocolate or strawberry	12 fl. oz.	8.0	5.0	2.0
Vanilla	12 fl. oz.	9.0	6.0	3.0
Syrup	1.5-oz. serving	Tr.	Tr.	Tr.
Turkey club	7.3-oz. serving	16.0	4.0	11.0
HAWAIIAN PUNCH, canned, regular or dietetic	6 fl. oz.	0.0		
HEADCHEESE (Oscar Mayer)	1-oz. slice	4.1		
HEART (USDA):				
Beef, lean, braised	4 oz.	6.5		
Calf, braised	4 oz.	10.3		
Chicken:				
Simmered	1 heart (5 grams)	.4		
Simmered, chopped or diced	1 cup (5.1 oz.)	10.4		

FOOD DESCRIPTION	MEASURE OR QUANTITY	FATS IN GRAMS		
		Total	Saturated	Unsaturated
Hog, braised	4 oz.	7.8		
Lamb, braised	4 oz.	16.3		
Turkey:				
Simmered	4 oz.	15.0		
Simmered, chopped or diced	1 cup (5.1 oz.)	19.1		
HEARTWISE, cereal (Kellogg's)	2/3 cup (1 oz.)	1.0		
HERRING (USDA):				
Raw:				
Atlantic, meat only	4 oz.	12.8	2.0	11.0
Pacific, meat only	4 oz.	2.9		
Canned, plain, solids & liq.	4 oz.	15.4		
Pickled, Bismarck type	4 oz.	17.1		
Salted or brined	4 oz.	17.2		
Smoked:				
Bloaters	4 oz.	14.1		
Hard	4 oz.	17.9		
Kippered	4 oz.	14.6		
HICKORY NUT (USDA) shelled	4 oz.	77.9	7.0	71.0
HOMINY GRITS:				
Dry:				
Degermed (USDA)	1/2 cup (2.8 oz.)	.6		
Instant (Quaker)	.8-oz. packet	.1		
Cooked (Albers)	1 cup	.2		
HONEY, strained (USDA)	Any quantity	0.0		
HONEYCOMB, cereal (Post)	1 1/3 cups (1 oz.)	.5		
HONEYDEW, fresh (USDA):				
Wedge	2″ × 7″ wedge (5.3 oz.)	.3		
Flesh only	4 oz.	.3		
HONEY SMACKS, cereal (Kellogg's)	3/4 cup	0.0		
HORSERADISH:				
Raw (USDA) pared	1 oz.	Tr.		
Dehydrated (Heinz)	1 T.	.2		
Prepared (USDA)	1 oz.	Tr.		
HOT BITES , frozen (Banquet):				
Cheese, mozzarella nuggets	1/4 of 10 1/2-oz. pkg.	13.0		
Chicken:				
Regular:				
Breast patties	1/4 of 10.5-oz. pkg.	13.0		
Breast tender, southern fried	1/4 of 10.5-oz. pkg.	7.0		
Drum snackers	1/4 of 10.5-oz. pkg.	15.0		
Nuggets:				
Plain or southern fried	1/4 of 10.5-oz. pkg.	14.0		
Hot & spicy	1/4 of 10.5-oz. pkg.	19.0		
Microwave:				
Breast pattie, regular or southern fried	4-oz. pkg.	14.0		
Breast tenders	4-oz. pkg.	10.0		
HOT WHEELS , cereal (Ralston-Purina)	1 cup (1 oz.)	1.0		
HYACINTH BEAN (USDA):				
Young pod, raw, trimmed	4 oz.	.3		
Dry seeds	4 oz.	1.7		
ICE CREAM (Listed by type, such as sandwich, or *Whammy,* or by flavor. See also **FROZEN DESSERT**):				
Almond amaretto (Baskin-Robbins)	4 fl. oz.	17.0		
Bar:				
(Good Humor) vanilla, chocolate-coated	3-fl.-oz. piece	11.0		
(Häagen-Dazs):				
Chocolate, dark-chocolate coating	1 bar	25.0		

FOOD DESCRIPTION	MEASURE OR QUANTITY	FATS IN GRAMS		
		Total	Saturated	Unsaturated
Vanilla, milk-chocolate coating	1 bar	23.0		
Butter pecan:				
(Good Humor)	4 fl. oz.	9.0		
(Häagen-Dazs)	4 fl. oz.	24.0		
Cappuccino:				
(Baskin-Robbins) chip	4 fl. oz.	19.0		
(Häagen-Dazs)	4 fl. oz.	16.0		
Chocolate:				
(Baskin-Robbins) regular	4 fl. oz.	12.6		
(Good Humor) bulk	4 fl. oz.	7.0		
(Häagen-Dazs) mint	4 fl. oz.	20.0		
Chocolate chip (Häagen-Dazs)	4 fl. oz.	18.0		
Chocolate eclair (Good Humor)	3-fl.-oz. piece	9.0		
Chocolate malt bar (Good Humor)	3-fl.-oz. piece	13.0		
Coffee (Häagen-Dazs) chip	4 fl. oz.	18.0		
Cookies & cream (Häagen-Dazs)	4 fl. oz.	17.2		
Cookie sandwich (Good Humor)	2.7-fl.-oz. piece	11.0		
Grand marnier (Baskin-Robbins)	4 fl. oz.	12.0		
Honey (Häagen-Dazs)	4 fl. oz.	16.9		
Macadamia nut (Häagen-Dazs)	4 fl. oz.	24.0		
Maple walnut (Häagen-Dazs)	4 fl. oz.	25.2		
Oreo, cookies 'n cream:				
Bulk	3 fl. oz.	8.0		
Sandwich	1 piece	11.0		
Pralines 'n cream (Baskin-Robbins)	1 scoop (2.5 fl. oz.)	13.1		
Rocky road (Baskin-Robbins)	4 fl. oz.	11.2		
Strawberry:				
(Baskin-Robbins) wild	4 fl. oz.	1.2		
(Häagen-Dazs)	4 fl. oz.	15.2		
Toasted almond bar (Good Humor)	3-fl.-oz. piece	8.0		
Vanilla:				
(Baskin-Robbins) regular	4 fl. oz.	13.1		
(Häagen-Dazs)	4 fl. oz.	17.0	10.0	5.7
(Meadow Gold)	½ cup	7.0		
Vanilla slice (Good Humor):				
Regular	3.2-fl.-oz. slice	6.1		
Calorie controlled	3.2-fl.-oz. slice	1.0		
Vanilla swiss almond (Häagen-Dazs)	4 fl. oz.	22.0		
Whammy (Good Humor) assorted	1.6-oz. piece	6.0		
ICE CREAM CONE, cone only (Baskin-Robbins):				
Cake	1 cone	.3		
Sugar	1 cone	1.0		
(Comet) sugar	1 cone	0.0		
ICE CREAM CUP, cup only				
(Comet) regular or chocolate	1 cup	0.0		
*ICE CREAM MIX (Salada) any flavor	1 cup	19.0		
ICE MILK:				
(USDA):				
Hardened	1 cup (4.6 oz.)	6.7	4.0	3.0
Soft serve	1 cup (6.2 oz.)	8.9	3.0	4.0
(Land O'Lakes) vanilla	4 fl. oz.	3.0	2.0	<2.0
(Weight Watchers) Grand Collection:				
Chocolate:				
Regular, fudge or swirl	½ cup	3.0	2.0	0.0
Chip	½ cup	4.0	2.0	0.0

FOOD DESCRIPTION	MEASURE OR QUANTITY	FATS IN GRAMS		
		Total	Saturated	Unsaturated
Neapolitan, strawberries & cream, or vanilla	½ cup	3.0	1.0	0.0
ICE TEASERS (Nestlé)	8 fl. oz.	0.0		
ICING (See **CAKE ICING**)				
INSTANT BREAKFAST (See individual brand name or company listings)				
IRISH WHISKEY (See **DISTILLED LIQUOR**)				
JACK IN THE BOX:				
Breakfast Jack	4.4-oz. serving	13.0		
Canadian crescent	4.7-oz. serving	31.0		
Cheesecake	3.5-oz. serving	17.5		
Chicken strips	1 piece	3.5		
Chicken supreme sandwich	8.1-oz. serving	36.0		
Club pita sandwich, excluding sauce	6.3-oz. serving	8.0		
Egg, scrambled, platter	8.8-oz. serving	40.0		
Egg roll	1 piece	6.3		
Fish supreme sandwich	8-oz. sandwich	32.0		
French fries:				
Regular	2.4-oz. order	12.0		
Jumbo	4.8-oz. order	24.0		
Hamburger:				
Regular	3.6-oz. serving	13.0		
Cheeseburger:				
Regular	4-oz. serving	14.0		
Bacon	8.1-oz. serving	39.0		
Ultimate	9.9-oz. serving	69.0		
Ham & swiss	9.1-oz. serving	49.0		
Jumbo Jack:				
Regular	7.8-oz. serving	34.0		
With cheese	8.5-oz. serving	40.0		
Monterey Burger	9.9-oz. serving	57.0		
Mushroom	6.4-oz. serving	47.0		
Swiss & bacon	6.6-oz. serving	47.0		
Milk shake:				
Chocolate or strawberry	11.4-oz. serving	7.0		
Vanilla	11.2-oz. serving	6.0		
Nachos:				
Cheese	6-oz. serving	35.0		
Supreme	11.9-oz. serving	45.0		
Onion rings	3.8-oz. serving	23.0		
Orange juice	6.5-oz. serving	0.0		
Pancake platter	8.1-oz. serving	22.0		
Salad:				
Chef	11.7-oz. salad	18.0		
Side	3.9-oz. salad	3.0		
Taco	14.8-oz. salad	38.0		
Salad dressing:				
Regular:				
Blue cheese	1.2-oz. serving	11.0		
Buttermilk	1.2-oz. serving	18.0		
Thousand island	1.2-oz. serving	15.0		
Dietetic or low-calorie, French	1.2-oz. serving	4.0		
Sauce:				
A-1	1.8-oz. serving	Tr.		
Barbecue or salsa	.9-oz. serving	Tr.		
Guacamole	.9-oz. serving	5.0		
Mayo-mustard	.8-oz. serving	13.0		
Mayo-onion	.8-oz. serving	15.0		
Seafood cocktail or sweet & sour	1-oz. serving	Tr.		
Sausage crescent	5.5-oz. serving	43.0		
Shrimp	1 piece (.3 oz.)	1.6		
Soft drink, sweetened or dietetic	12 fl. oz.	0.0		
Supreme crescent	5.1-oz. serving	40.0		
Syrup, pancake	1.5-oz. serving	0.0		

FOOD DESCRIPTION	MEASURE OR QUANTITY	FATS IN GRAMS Total	Saturated	Unsaturated
Taco:				
Regular	2.9-oz. serving	11.0		
Super	4.8-oz. serving	17.0		
Turnover, hot apple	4.2-oz. piece	24.0		
JACK MACKEREL, raw, meat only (USDA)	4 oz.	6.4		
JAM, SWEETENED (See also individual listings by flavor) (USDA)	1 T. (.7 oz.)	Tr.		
JELLY, sweetened (See also individual listings by flavor) (USDA)	1 T. (.6 oz.)	Tr.		
JELL-O FRUIT & CREAM BAR, any flavor	1.7-oz. bar	2.8		
JELL-O PUDDING POPS, any flavor	2-oz. bar	2.6		
JERUSALEM ARTICHOKE (USDA) Pared	4 oz.	.1		
JUICE (See individual listings)				
JUJUBE OR CHINESE DATE (USDA):				
Fresh, flesh only	4 oz.	.2		
Dried, flesh only	1 oz.	.3		
JUST RIGHT, cereal (Kellogg's)	2/3 cup (1 oz.)	1.0		
KABOOMS, cereal (General Mills)	1 cup (1 oz.)	6.0		
KALE:				
Raw (USDA) leaves including stems	1 lb. (weighed trimmed)	2.7		
Boiled (USDA) leaves including stems	1/2 cup (1.9 oz.)	.4		
Canned (Allen) chopped, solids & liq.	1/2 cup	Tr.		
Frozen, chopped:				
(Birds Eye)	1/3 of 10-oz. pkg.	.4		
(McKenzie)	3.3 oz.	0.0		
KENMEI, cereal:				
Plain	3/4 cup (1 oz.)	1.0		
Almond & raisin	3/4 cup (1.4 oz.)	2.0		
KENTUCKY FRIED CHICKEN:				
Biscuit, buttermilk	2.3-oz. serving	11.7	2.2	3.2
Chicken:				
Original recipe:				
Breast:				
Center	4-oz. piece	15.3		
Side	3.2-oz. piece	16.5		
Drumstick	2-oz. piece	8.5		
Thigh	3.7-oz. piece	19.7		
Wing	1.9-oz. piece	11.7		
Extra tasty crispy:				
Breast:				
Center	4.8-oz. piece	19.7		
Side	3.7-oz. piece	22.3		
Drumstick	2.4-oz. piece	13.9		
Thigh	4.2-oz. piece	29.8		
Wing	2.3-oz. piece	18.6		
Lite 'n Crispy:				
Breast:				
Center	3-oz. serving	11.9		
Side	2.6-oz. serving	12.4		
Drumstick	1.7-oz. serving	7.0		
Thigh	2.8-oz. serving	16.7		
Chicken Littles, sandwich	1.7-oz. serving	10.1		
Chicken nugget	.6-oz. piece	2.9		
Chicken sandwich, *Colonel's*	5.9-oz. sandwich	27.3		
Corn on the cob	5-oz. serving	3.1		

FOOD DESCRIPTION	MEASURE OR QUANTITY	FATS IN GRAMS		
		Total	Saturated	Unsaturated
Hot wings	.7-oz. piece	4.0		
Potatoes:				
French fries	2.7-oz. serving	11.9		
⌐ Mashed, & gravy	3.5-oz. serving	1.6		
Sauce:				
Barbecue or Sweet & Sour	1-oz. serving	.6		
Honey	.5-oz. serving	Tr.		
Mustard	1-oz. serving	.9		
KETCHUP (See **CATSUP**)				
KIDNEY (USDA):				
Beef, braised	4 oz.	13.6		
Calf, raw	4 oz.	5.2		
Hog, raw	4 oz.	4.1		
Lamb, raw	4 oz.	3.7		
KIPPERS (See **HERRING**)				
KIX, cereal (General Mills)	1½ cups (1 oz.)	Tr.		
KOHLRABI (USDA) boiled, drained	1 cup (5.5 oz.)	.2		
KOOL-AID (General Foods), regular or sugar sweetened	1 cup	Tr.		
KRISPIES, cereal (Kellogg's)	Any quantity	0.0		
KUMQUAT, fresh (USDA) flesh & skin	4 oz.	.1		
LAKE HERRING, raw (USDA) meat only	4 oz.	2.6		
LAKE TROUT, raw (USDA) meat only	4 oz.	11.3		
LAMB, choice grade (USDA):				
Chop, broiled:				
Loin. One 5-oz. chop (weighed with bone before cooking) will give you:				
Lean & fat	2.8 oz.	22.9	13.0	10.0
Lean only	2.3 oz.	4.9	3.0	2.0
Rib. One 5-oz. chop (weighed with bone before cooking) will give you:				
Lean & fat	2.9 oz.	29.2	16.0	13.0
Lean only	2 oz.	5.9	3.0	3.0
Fat, separable, cooked	1 oz.	21.4	12.0	10.0
Leg:				
Raw, lean & fat	1 lb. (weighed with bone)	61.7	35.0	27.0
Roasted:				
Lean & fat	4 oz.	21.4	12.0	9.0
Lean only	4 oz.	7.9	4.0	4.0
Shoulder:				
Raw, lean & fat	1 lb. (weighed with bone)	92.0	52.0	40.0
Roasted:				
Lean & fat	4 oz.	30.8	17.0	14.0
Lean only	4 oz.	11.3	6.0	5.0
LAMB'S QUARTERS (USDA) boiled, drained	4 oz.	.8		
LARD (See **FAT, COOKING**)				
LASAGNE:				
Canned (Hormel) *Short Orders*	7½-oz. can	14.0		
Frozen:				
(Banquet) *Family Entrees,* with meat sauce	32-oz. pkg.	40.0		
(Buitoni):				
Cheese, sorrentino	8-oz. serving	9.1	4.7	2.7
With meat sauce	5-oz. serving	8.3	4.6	3.0
(Celentano):				
Regular	½ of 16-oz. pkg.	19.0		
Primavera	11-oz. pkg.	14.0		
(Healthy Choice) with meat sauce	9-oz. meal	5.0	2.0	1.0

FOOD DESCRIPTION	MEASURE OR QUANTITY	FATS IN GRAMS		
		Total	Saturated	Unsaturated
(Stouffer's):				
Regular:				
Plain	10½-oz. serving	13.0		
Vegetable	10½-oz. serving	24.0		
Lean Cuisine, meat sauce	10¼-oz. serving	8.0		
(Weight Watchers):				
Garden	11-oz. meal	12.0	5.0	7.0
Italian cheese	11-oz. meal	14.0	7.0	7.0
Meat sauce	11-oz. meal	11.0	5.0	6.0
LEEKS, raw (USDA) trimmed	4 oz.	.3		
LEMON, fresh (USDA):				
Fruit, including peel	1 lb. (weighed whole)	1.3		
Peeled fruit	1 med. lemon (2⅛")	.2		
LEMONADE:				
Canned:				
Capri Sun	6¾ fl. oz.	0.0		
(Hi-C)	6 fl. oz.	Tr.		
Chilled (Minute Maid)	6 fl. oz.	Tr.		
*Frozen, *Country Time*	8 fl. oz.	Tr.		
*Mix, regular, *Country Time*, presweetened	8 fl. oz.	Tr.		
LEMON JUICE:				
Fresh (USDA)	1 T. (.5 oz.)	Tr.		
Plastic container (ReaLemon)	1 T. (.5 oz.)	Tr.		
Frozen, unsweetened:				
Concentrate (USDA)	½ cup (5.1 oz.)	1.3		
Single strength (USDA)	½ cup (4.3 oz.)	.2		
Full strength, already recon- stituted (Minute Maid)	½ cup (4.2 oz.)	Tr.		
LEMON PEEL, raw or candied (USDA)	1 oz.	Tr.		
LEMON PIE (See **PIE,** Lemon)				
LENTIL:				
Whole (USDA):				
Dry	1 cup (6.7 oz.)	2.1		
Cooked, drained	½ cup (3.6 oz.)	Tr.		
Split, dry, without seed coat (USDA)	½ lb.	2.0		
LETTUCE (USDA):				
Bibb or Boston, untrimmed	7.8-oz. head (4" dia.)	.3		
Cos (See Romaine)				
Grand Rapids	2 large leaves (1.8 oz.)	.2		
Iceberg, leaves, chopped or chunks	1 cup	Tr.		
Romaine:				
Untrimmed	1 lb. (weighed untrimmed)	.9		
Shredded & broken into pieces	½ cup (.8 oz.)	Tr.		
Salad Bowl, trimmed	2 large leaves (1.8 oz.)	.2		
LIME, fresh, whole (USDA)	1 med. (2" dia., 2.4 oz.)	.1		
LIMEADE, concentrate, sweet- ened, frozen:				
*Diluted with 4⅓ parts water (USDA)	½ cup (4.4 oz.)	Tr.		
(ReaLemon)	6-oz. can	.2		
LIME ICE, home recipe (USDA)	8 oz. (by wt.)	Tr.		
LIME JUICE:				
Fresh (USDA)	1 cup (8.7 oz.)	.2		
(Rose's)	1 fl. oz.	0.0		
LINGCOD, raw (USDA) meat only	4 oz.	.9		
LINGUINI, frozen:				
(Healthy Choice) with shrimp	9½-oz. meal	2.0	1.0	1.0
(Stouffer's) *Lean Cuisine*, with clam sauce	9⅝-oz. meal	7.0		
(Weight Watchers) seafood	9-oz. meal	7.0	1.0	6.0
LITCHI NUT (USDA):				
Fresh, flesh only	4 oz.	.3		
Dried, flesh only	2 oz.	.7		

FOOD DESCRIPTION	MEASURE OR QUANTITY	FATS IN GRAMS		
		Total	Saturated	Unsaturated
LIVER (USDA):				
Beef, fried	4 oz.	12.0		
Calf, fried	4 oz.	15.0		
Chicken, simmered	4 oz.	5.0		
Goose, raw	1 lb.	45.4		
Hog, fried	4 oz.	13.0		
Lamb, broiled	4 oz.	14.1		
Turkey, simmered	4 oz.	5.4		
LIVER SAUSAGE OR LIVER-WURST:				
Fresh (USDA)	1 oz.	7.3		
Packaged (Oscar Mayer):				
Sliced	.9-oz. slice	8.8		
Ring	1 oz.	7.9		
Smoked (USDA)	1 oz.	7.8		
LIVERWURST SPREAD:				
(Hormel)	1 oz.	6.0		
(Underwood)	1 oz.	7.9		
LOBSTER (USDA):				
Raw, meat only	4 oz.	2.2		
Cooked, meat only	4 oz.	1.7		
Canned, meat only	4 oz.	1.7		
LOBSTER NEWBURG, home recipe (USDA)	1 cup (8.8 oz.)	26.5		
LOBSTER PASTE, canned (USDA)	1 oz.	2.7		
LOBSTER SALAD, home recipe (USDA)	4 oz.	7.3		
LOGANBERRY (USDA):				
Fresh, trimmed	1 cup (5.1 oz.)	.9		
Canned, solids & liq.:				
Water pack, light, heavy or extra heavy syrup	4 oz.	.5		
Juice pack	4 oz.	.6		
LONG JOHN SILVER'S :				
Catfish:				
Dinner	13.2-oz. serving	42.0	36.0	6.1
Fillet	2½-oz. piece	11.0	10.1	.8
Catsup	.4-oz. packet	Tr.		
Chicken Plank:				
Dinner:				
3-piece	13-oz. dinner	39.0	5.1	33.4
4-piece	14.6-oz. dinner	44.0	5.3	39.0
Single piece	1.6-oz. piece	6.0	.2	5.7
Children's meals:				
Chicken Planks	7.1-oz. meal	24.0	.9	22.8
Fish	6½-oz. meal	20.0	.8	19.0
Fish & chicken planks	8.1-oz. meal	26.0	1.0	24.6
Chowder, clam with cod	7-oz. serving	6.0	1.7	4.3
Clam:				
Breaded	2.3-oz. serving	12.0	.6	10.6
Dinner	12.8-oz. meal	45.0	5.7	39.4
Cod, entree:				
Baked:				
Regular	5.8-oz. serving	Tr.		
Delight	6-oz. meal	1.0		
Supreme	6.2-oz. meal	4.0		
Broiled	5.4-oz. serving	2.0		
Corn on the cob, with whirl	6.6-oz. serving	14.0	3.5	8.4
Fish, battered	2.6-oz. piece	8.0	.3	7.6
Fish & chicken entree	14-oz. serving	40.0	5.2	35.2
Fish dinner, 3-piece	16.1-oz. serving	44.0	38.8	5.4
Fish dinner, home-style:				
3-piece	13.1-oz. meal	42.0	9.5	32.6
4-piece	14.8-oz. meal	50.0	11.9	38.0
6-piece	18.1-oz. meal	64.0	14.3	48.8
Fish & fryes, entree:				
2-piece	10-oz. meal	30.0	7.3	24.7
3-piece	12.6-oz. meal	38.0	9.1	28.6
Fish, homestyle	1.6-oz. piece	7.0	1.6	5.9

FOOD DESCRIPTION	MEASURE OR QUANTITY	FATS IN GRAMS		
		Total	Saturated	Unsaturated
Fish & more, entree	13.4-oz. meal	37.0	8.3	28.2
Fish sandwich, homestyle	6.9-oz. serving	22.0	4.9	16.6
Fish sandwich platter, home-style	13.4-oz. meal	38.0	8.4	29.2
Hushpuppie	.8-oz. piece	2.0	.4	1.5
Pie:				
Lemon meringue	4.2-oz. slice	7.0	2.5	4.4
Pecan	4.4-oz. slice	25.0	7.2	17.6
Potato:				
Baked, without topping	7.1-oz. serving	Tr.		
Fryes	3-oz. order	10.0	2.6	7.3
Rice pilaf	3-oz. serving	2.0		
Roll, dinner, plain	.9-oz. piece	1.0		
Salad:				
Garden	8.7-oz. serving	9.0		
Ocean chef	11.3-oz. serving	9.0		
Seafood, entree	11.9-oz. serving	7.0	.8	4.5
Side	4.3-oz. serving	Tr.		
Salad dressing:				
Regular:				
Bleu cheese	1.5-oz. packet	2.0	.5	1.5
Ranch	1.5-oz. packet	3.0	.5	2.5
Sea salad	1.6-oz. packet	7.0	2.8	4.3
Dietetic, Italian	1.6-oz. serving	1.0	.4	.7
Salmon, broiled	4.4-oz. piece	4.0		
Sauce:				
Honey mustard	1.2-oz. packet	Tr.	Tr.	Tr.
Seafood	1.2-oz. packet	1.0	.3	.7
Sweet & sour	1.2-oz. packet	Tr.	Tr.	Tr.
Tartar	1-oz. packet	3.0	.6	2.3
Seafood platter, entree	14.1-oz. serving	46.0	10.3	35.7
Shrimp, battered	.5-oz. piece	3.0	.7	2.3
Shrimp, breaded	2.2-oz. serving	10.0	2.3	7.7
Shrimp dinner, battered:				
6-piece	11.1-oz. meal	37.0	8.3	28.4
9-piece	12.5-oz. meal	45.0	10.1	34.4
Shrimp feast, breaded:				
13-piece	12.56-oz. serving	41.0	9.1	31.4
21-piece	14.8-oz. serving	51.0	11.3	38.9
Shrimp, fish & chicken dinner	13.4-oz. serving	40.0	9.1	30.7
Shrimp & fish dinner	12.3-oz. serving	37.0	8.3	28.2
Shrimp scampi, baked, entree	5.7-oz. serving	7.0		
Vegetables, mixed	4-oz. serving	2.0	.6	1.4
Vinegar, malt	.4-oz. packet	Tr.		
LOQUAT, fresh (USDA) flesh only	4 oz.	.2		
LUCKY CHARMS, cereal (General Mills)	1 cup (1 oz.)	1.0		
LUNCHEON MEAT (See also individual listings, e.g., **BOLOGNA**):				
All meat (Oscar Mayer)	1-oz. slice	8.6	3.4	5.5
Barbecue loaf (Oscar Mayer)	1-oz. slice	2.5	1.0	1.4
Gourmet loaf (Eckrich)	1 slice	1.0		
Honey loaf (Oscar Mayer)	1-oz. slice	1.0	.7	.7
Liver cheese (Oscar Mayer)	1-oz. slice	10.0	3.5	6.2
Macaroni & cheese loaf (Eckrich)	1-oz. slice	6.0		
Meat loaf (USDA)	1 oz.	3.7		
New England brand (Oscar Mayer)	1-oz. slice	1.3	.6	1.1
Old-fashioned loaf:				
(Eckrich)	1-oz. slice	6.0		
(Oscar Mayer)	1-oz. slice	4.0	1.6	2.6
Olive loaf:				
(Eckrich)	1-oz. slice	7.0		
(Oscar Mayer)	1-oz. slice	3.9	1.5	2.6
Peppered loaf (Oscar Mayer)	1-oz. slice	1.5	.8	1.2
Pickle & pimiento loaf (Oscar Mayer)	1-oz. slice	3.9	1.5	2.5

FOOD DESCRIPTION	MEASURE OR QUANTITY	FATS IN GRAMS		
		Total	Saturated	Unsaturated
LUNG, raw (USDA):				
Beef or lamb	1 lb.	10.4		
Calf	1 lb.	17.2		
MACADAMIA NUT (USDA)				
shelled	4 oz.	81.2		
MACARONI. Plain macaroni products are essentially the same in caloric value and carbohydrate content on the same weight basis. The longer they are cooked, the more water is absorbed and this affects the nutritive values.				
Dry (USDA)	1 oz.	.3		
Cooked (USDA)	4 oz.	.6		
Canned (Franco-American):				
BeefyOs, & beef in tomato sauce	7½-oz. can	8.0		
PizzOs, in pizza sauce	7½-oz. can	2.0		
Frozen, & beef:				
(Stouffer's) with tomatoes	½ of 11½-oz. pkg.	8.0		
(Swanson)	12-oz. dinner	14.0		
MACARONI & CHEESE:				
Home recipe, baked (USDA)	1 cup (7.1 oz.)	22.2	10.0	12.0
Canned:				
(USDA)	1 cup (8.5 oz.)	9.6	5.0	5.0
(Franco-American)	7⅜-oz. can	5.0		
Frozen:				
(Banquet):				
Casserole	8-oz. meal	17.0		
Dinner	10-oz. meal	20.0		
(Birds Eye) classics	½ of 10-oz. pkg.	11.0		
(Celentano) baked	½ of 11-oz. pkg.	13.0		
(Green Giant) one serving	5½-oz. pkg.	9.0	4.0	Tr.
MACARONI&CHEESEPIE, frozen (Swanson)	7-oz. pie	9.0		
MACKEREL (USDA):				
Atlantic:				
Raw, meat only	4 oz.	13.8		
Broiled with butter, margarine or vegetable shortening	8½" × 2½" × ½" fillet (3.7 oz.)	16.6		
Canned, solids & liq.	4 oz.	12.6		
Pacific:				
Raw, meat only	4 oz.	8.3		
Canned, solids & liq.	4 oz.	11.3		
Salted	4 oz.	28.5		
Smoked	4 oz.	14.7		
MACKEREL, JACK (See **JACK MACKEREL**)				
MAI TAI COCKTAIL MIX (Holland House)	.6-oz. serving	0.0		
MALT, dry (USDA)	1 oz.	.5		
MALTED MILK MIX:				
(USDA):				
Dry powder, "unfortified"	1 oz. (3 heaping tsps.)	2.4		
*Prepared with whole milk	1 cup (8.3 oz.)	10.3		
(Carnation) chocolate	3 heaping tsps. (.7 oz.)	1.7	Tr.	Tr.
MALT LIQUOR	Any quantity	0.0		
MALT-O-MEAL, cereal	1 T.	0.0		
MAMEY OR MAMMEE APPLE, fresh (USDA) flesh only	4 oz.	.6		
MANDARIN ORANGE, FRESH (See **TANGERINE**)				
MANGO, fresh (USDA):				
Whole	1 med. (7.1 oz.)	.5		
Flesh only, diced or sliced	½ cup (2.9 oz.)	3.0		

FOOD DESCRIPTION	MEASURE OR QUANTITY	FATS IN GRAMS		
		Total	Saturated	Unsaturated
MANICOTTI, frozen:				
(Celentano)	10-oz. pkg.	14.0		
(Weight Watchers) cheese	9¼-oz. meal	13.0	5.0	7.0
MANWICH (Hunt's):				
Original	5.8-oz. serving	13.0		
Mexican flavor	5.8-oz. serving	14.0		
MAPLE SYRUP (See **SYRUP,** Maple)				
MARGARINE:				
Regular, salted or unsalted:				
(Blue Bonnet)	1 T.	11.0		
(Fleischmann's)	1 T.	11.0		
I Can't Believe It's Not Butter, soft, tub or squeezable	1 T.	10.0		
(Imperial) soft or stick	1 T.	11.0		
(Land O'Lakes) stick or tub	1 T.	12.0	3.0	9.0
(Mazola)	1 T.	11.2	1.9	9.1
Nucoa	1 T.	11.2	2.1	9.0
(Promise) soft or stick	1 T.	10.0	4.0	5.0
(Shedd's):				
Regular	1 T.	7.0		
Country Crock:				
Soft	1 T.	7.0		
Stick	1 T.	9.0		
Squeezable	1 T.	9.0		
Imitation or dietetic:				
Country Morning:				
Regular, stick	1 T.	12.0	3.0	9.0
Light, tub	1 T.	9.0	3.0	6.0
(Imperial) diet or light	1 T.	6.0	1.0	3.0
(Land O'Lakes):				
Made with soy oil spread, 64%, tub	1 T.	9.0	3.0	6.0
Made with sweet cream:				
Stick	1 T.	12.0	3.0	9.0
Tub	1 T.	9.0	3.0	6.0
Mazola	1 T.	5.5	.9	4.5
(Promise):				
Light, soft or stick	1 T.	7.0		
Extra light, soft	1 T.	6.0		
(Weight Watchers):				
Regular, reduced calorie	1 T. (.5 oz.)	7.0	1.0	3.0
Made with corn oil, light spread or sweet	1 T.	6.0	1.0	3.0
Whipped:				
(Blue Bonnet):				
Spread, 60% fat	1 T.	6.0		
Stick	1 T.	7.0		
(Fleischmann's)	1 T.	7.0		
(Imperial) spread	1 T.	4.0		
MARGARITA COCKTAIL MIX (Holland House)	Any quantity	0.0		
MARINADE MIX, MEAT:				
(French's)	1-oz. pkg.	0.0		
(Kikkoman)	1-oz. pkg.	.4		
MARMALADE:				
Sweetened (Smucker's)	1 T.	Tr.		
Low-calorie (Estee)	1 T.	0.0		
MARSHMALLOW FLUFF	1 heaping tsp.	.1		
MATZO (Manischewitz):				
Regular:				
Plain	1-oz. piece	3.0		
American	1-oz. board	1.2		
Egg	1 matzo	2.0		
Miniature	2-gram matzo	Tr.		
Tea, thin	1 matzo	.3		
Tam Tam, any flavor	1 matzo	.8		

FOOD DESCRIPTION	MEASURE OR QUANTITY	FATS IN GRAMS		
		Total	Saturated	Unsaturated
Dietetic:				
Tam Tam, unsalted	1 piece	.7		
Thins	1 piece	.4		
MATZO FARFEL (Manische-witz)	½ cup	.4		
MATZO MEAL (Manischewitz)	1 cup (4.1 oz.)	.9	0.0	.7
MAYONNAISE:				
Regular:				
(USDA)	1 cup (7.8 oz.)	176.5	31.0	146.0
(USDA)	1 T. (.5 oz.)	11.2	2.0	9.0
(Hellmann's)	1 T.	11.0		
Imitation:				
Heart Beat (GFA)	1 T.	4.0	Tr.	2.0
(Weight Watchers)	1 T.	5.0	1.0	3.0
McDONALD'S:				
Big Mac	1 hamburger	35.0		
Biscuit:				
Plain	1 serving	18.2		
With bacon, egg & cheese	1 serving	31.6		
With sausage	1 serving	30.9		
With sausage & egg	1 serving	39.9		
Cheeseburger	1 serving	16.0		
Chicken McNuggets	1 serving	21.3		
Chicken McNuggets sauce:				
Barbecue	1.1-oz. serving	.4		
Honey	.5-oz. serving	Tr.		
Hot mustard	1.1-oz. serving	2.4		
Cookies:				
Chocolate chip	1 package	16.3		
McDonaldland	1 package	10.8		
Egg McMuffin	1 serving	15.8		
Egg, scrambled	1 serving	13.0		
English muffin, with butter	1 serving	5.3		
Filet-O-Fish	1 sandwich	25.7		
Grapefruit juice	6 fl. oz.	.2		
Hamburger	1 serving	11.3		
Hot cakes with butter & syrup	1 serving	10.3		
McLean Deluxe	1 serving	10.0	4.0	6.0
Pie:				
Apple	1 serving	14.3		
Cherry	1 serving	13.6		
Potato:				
Fries	1 regular order	11.5		
Hash browns	1 order	7.0		
Quarter Pounder:				
Regular	1 hamburger	23.5		
With cheese	1 hamburger	31.6		
Salad:				
Chef's	1 serving	13.6	5.9	7.6
Chicken oriental	1 serving	3.4	.9	2.4
Garden	1 serving	6.8	2.9	3.9
Shrimp	1 serving	2.8	.7	2.1
Side	1 serving	4.1	1.6	2.4
Salad dressing:				
Regular:				
Blue cheese	.5 oz.	6.9		
French	.5 oz.	5.2		
Oriental	.5 oz.	.1		
Thousand island	.5 oz.	7.5		
Dietetic, vinaigrette	.5 oz.	.5		
Sausage McMuffin:				
Plain	1 sandwich	21.9	7.8	14.1
With egg	1 sandwich	27.4		
Sausage, pork	1 serving	16.3	5.9	10.4
Shake:				
Chocolate	1 serving	10.6		
Strawberry	1 serving	10.1		
Vanilla	1 serving	10.2		

FOOD DESCRIPTION	MEASURE OR QUANTITY	FATS IN GRAMS		
		Total	Saturated	Unsaturated
Sundae:				
Caramel, hot	1 serving	9.1		
Hot fudge	1 serving	9.4		
Strawberry	1 serving	7.3		
MEAL (See **CORNMEAL, CRACKER MEAL** or **MATZO MEAL**)				
MEATBALL DINNER OR ENTREE:				
*Canned (Hunt's) *Minute Gourmet*	7.6-oz. serving	18.0		
Frozen (Swanson)	8½-oz. meal	18.0		
MEATBALL STEW, frozen (Stouffer's) *Lean Cuisine*	10-oz. serving	10.0		
MEATBALLS, SWEDISH, frozen:				
(Armour) *Dinner Classics*	11½-oz. meal	18.0		
(Stouffer's) with noodles	11-oz. pkg.	27.0		
MEAT LOAF DINNER, frozen:				
(Banquet) dinner	11-oz. dinner	27.0		
(Morton)	10-oz. dinner	17.3		
MEAT LOAF SEASONING MIX:				
*(Bell's)	4½-oz. pkg.	20.0		
(Contadina)	3¾-oz. pkg.	3.2		
MEAT, POTTED:				
(Hormel)	1 T.	2.0		
(Libby's)	⅓ of 5-oz. can	8.4		
MEAT TENDERIZER (French's) seasoned or unseasoned	1 tsp.	Tr.		
MELBA TOAST:				
(Keebler)	1 piece	Tr.		
(Old London)	1 piece	Tr.		
MELON (See individual listings, e.g., **CANTALOUPE, WATERMELON,** etc.)				
MELON BALL, in syrup, frozen (USDA)	½ cup (4.1 oz.)	.1		
MENUDO, canned (Old El Paso)	½ cup	52.0		
MEXICAN DINNER, frozen:				
(Banquet):				
Regular	12-oz. dinner	18.0		
Combination	12-oz. dinner	17.0		
(Patio):				
Regular	13¼-oz. meal	25.0		
Fiesta	12¼-oz. meal	20.0		
(Swanson):				
4-compartment meal	16-oz. meal	26.0		
Hungry-Man	22-oz. dinner	46.0		
MILK, CONDENSED, sweetened, canned:				
(USDA)	1 cup (10.8 oz.)	26.6	13.0	13.0
(Carnation)	1 fl. oz.	3.3		
MILK, DRY:				
Whole (USDA):				
Packed	1 cup (5.1 oz.)	39.9	22.0	18.0
Spooned	1 cup (4.3 oz.)	33.3	18.0	15.0
Nonfat, instant:				
(USDA)	⅞ cup dry (3.2 oz. dry makes 1 quart prepared)	.7		
*(Carnation)	1 cup (8.6 oz.)	.3	Tr.	Tr.
MILK, EVAPORATED, canned:				
Regular:				
(USDA) unsweetened	1 cup (8.9 oz.)	19.9	10.0	10.0
(Pet)	1 cup	20.0		
Skimmed (Carnation)	1 cup (9 oz.)	.5		

FOOD DESCRIPTION	MEASURE OR QUANTITY	FATS IN GRAMS		
		Total	Saturated	Unsaturated
MILK, FRESH:				
Whole:				
(USDA):				
3.5% fat	1 cup (8.6 oz.)	8.5	5.0	4.0
3.7% fat	1 cup (8.5 oz.)	8.9	5.0	4.0
(Borden's) regular or hi-calcium	1 cup	8.0		
(Johanna)	1 cup	8.0		
Buttermilk, cultured, fresh:				
(USDA)	1 cup (8.6 oz.)	.2		
(Friendship)	1 cup	4.0		
(Land O'Lakes)	8 fl. oz.	2.0		
Buttermilk, cultured, dried				
(USDA)	1 cup (4.2 oz.)	6.4	4.0	3.0
Chocolate milk drink, fresh:				
(USDA):				
With whole milk	1 cup (8.8 oz.)	8.5	4.0	5.0
With skim milk & 2% added butterfat	1 cup (8.8 oz.)	5.8	2.0	3.0
(Hershey's) 2% low-fat	1 cup (8 fl. oz.)	5.0		
(Johanna):				
Regular	1 cup	8.0		
Low-fat	1 cup	2.0		
(Land O'Lakes) low-fat:				
½% low-fat	8 fl. oz.	1.0	1.0	<2.0
Sweetened with *Nutra-sweet*	8 fl. oz.	3.0	2.0	<2.0
(Nestlé) *Quik*	8 fl. oz.	8.0		
Skim:				
(Borden's) regular or *Skimline*	1 cup	1.0		
(Land O'Lakes)	8 fl. oz.	1.0	<1.0	
(Weight Watchers)	1 cup	<1.0		
MILK, GOAT, whole (USDA)	1 cup (8.6 oz.)	9.8	5.0	5.0
MILK, HUMAN (USDA)	1 oz. (by wt.)	1.1	<1.0	<1.0
MINCEMEAT, (See **PIE FILLING,** Mincemeat)				
MINCE PIE (See **PIE,** Mince)				
MINERAL WATER	Any quantity	0.0		
MINI-WHEATS, cereal				
(Kellogg's) frosted	.25-oz. biscuit	0.0		
MOLASSES (Grandma's)	1 T.	0.0		
MOUSSE:				
Frozen (Weight Watchers):				
Chocolate or raspberry	½ of 5-oz. pkg.	6.0	<1.0	6.0
Praline pecan	½ of 5.4-oz. pkg.	7.0	1.0	6.0
*Mix:				
(Knorr):				
Unflavored	½ cup	5.0		
Chocolate:				
Dark or milk	½ cup	5.0		
White	½ cup	4.0		
(Estee) any flavor	½ cup	3.0	1.5	
Lite Whip (TKI Foods):				
Made with skim milk	½ cup	2.0		
Made with whole milk	½ cup	3.0		
MUESLIX, cereal (Kellogg's)	⅔ cup	2.0		
MUFFIN:				
Apple (Pepperidge Farm) with spice	1 muffin	8.0		
Blueberry:				
(USDA) home recipe	3″ muffin (1.4 oz.)	3.7	1.0	3.0
(Pepperidge Farm)	1.9-oz. muffin	7.0		
Bran:				
(USDA) home recipe	3″ muffin (1.4 oz.)	3.9	2.0	1.9
(Pepperidge Farm) with raisins	1 muffin	7.0		
Chocolate chip (Pepperidge Farm)	1 muffin	8.0		

FOOD DESCRIPTION	MEASURE OR QUANTITY	FATS IN GRAMS		
		Total	Saturated	Unsaturated
Corn:				
(USDA) home recipe, prepared with whole ground cornmeal	2⅜-oz. muffin	4.1	2.0	3.0
(Pepperidge Farm)	1.9-oz. muffin	7.0		
English:				
(Pepperidge Farm):				
Plain	2-oz. muffin	4.0		
Cinnamon raisin	2-oz. muffin	2.0		
(Roman Meal)	2-oz. muffin	.7		
(Thomas'):				
Regular or honey wheat	1 muffin	1.1		
Raisin	1 muffin	1.5		
MUFFIN MIX:				
*Apple cinnamon (Betty Crocker):				
Regular recipe	1/12 of pkg.	4.0	1.0	3.0
No-cholesterol recipe	1/12 of pkg.	3.0	1.0	2.0
*Banana, *Gold Medal*	1/6 of pkg.	5.0		
*Banana nut (Betty Crocker):				
Regular recipe	1/12 of pkg.	5.0	1.0	4.0
No-cholesterol recipe	1/12 of pkg.	4.0	1.0	3.0
Blueberry:				
*(Betty Crocker) wild:				
Regular recipe	1 muffin	4.0	1.0	3.0
No-cholesterol recipe	1 muffin	3.0	< 1.0	< 3.0
(Duncan Hines):				
Bakery-style	1/12 of pkg.	4.9		
Wild	1/12 of pkg.	2.7		
Gold Medal	1/6 of pkg.	6.0		
*Carrot nut (Betty Crocker) regular or no-cholesterol recipe	1/12 of pkg.	5.0	1.0	4.0
Cinnamon swirl (Duncan Hines) bakery-style	1/12 of pkg.	5.4		
*Corn (Dromedary)	1 muffin	4.0		
Cranberry orange nut (Duncan Hines) bakery-style	1/12 of pkg.	7.1		
*Honey bran, *Gold Medal*	1/6 of pkg.	6.0		
Oat bran:				
*(Betty Crocker):				
Regular recipe	1/8 of pkg.	8.0	2.0	6.0
No-cholesterol recipe	1/8 of pkg.	7.0	2.0	5.0
(Duncan Hines):				
Blueberry	1/12 of pkg.	3.1		
& honey	1/12 of pkg.	4.4		
Pecan nut (Duncan Hines)	1/12 of pkg.	9.7		
MULLET, raw (USDA) meat only	4 oz.	7.8		
MUNG BEAN SPROUT (See **BEAN SPROUT**)				
MUSHROOM:				
Raw (USDA):				
Whole	½ lb. (weighed untrimmed)	.6		
Trimmed, slices	½ cup (1.2 oz.)	.1		
Canned, solids & liq.:				
(USDA)	½ cup (4.3 oz.)	.1		
(B in B) sliced, chopped or whole, broiled in butter	6-oz. can	2.5		
Frozen (Birds Eye) whole	⅓ of 8-oz. pkg.	0.0		
MUSKRAT, roasted (USDA)	4 oz.	4.6		
MUSSEL (USDA):				
Raw, Atlantic & Pacific, meat only	4 oz.	2.5		
Canned, Pacific, drained	4 oz.	3.7		
MUSTARD, prepared:				
Brown (French's) spicy	1 tsp.	.3		
Chinese:				
(Chun King)	1 tsp.	.4		
(La Choy) hot	1 tsp.	< 1.0		

FOOD DESCRIPTION	MEASURE OR QUANTITY	FATS IN GRAMS		
		Total	Saturated	Unsaturated
GreyPoupon	1 tsp. (6 grams)	.3		
Horseradish (French's)	1 tsp.	.3		
Yellow (French's)	1 tsp.	.3		
MUSTARD GREENS:				
Raw, whole (USDA)	1 lb. (weighed untrimmed)	1.6		
Boiled without salt, drained (USDA)	1 cup (7.8 oz.)	.9		
Canned, solids & liq. (Sun-shine)	½ cup	.3		
Frozen:				
(Birds Eye) chopped	⅓ of 10-oz. pkg.	.2		
(Frosty Acres)	3.3 oz.	0.0		
MUSTARD SPINACH (USDA):				
Raw	1 lb.	1.4		
Boiled, drained	4 oz.	.2		
NATHAN'S:				
French fries	1 regular order	31.0		
Hamburger & roll	4½-oz. serving	23.0		
Hot dog & bun	1 serving	19.0		
NATURAL CEREAL:				
Familia:				
Regular	½ cup	2.9		
Bran	½ cup	3.4		
No added salt	½ cup	3.2		
Heartland (Pet):				
Regular, raisin or trail mix	¼ cup (1 oz.)	4.0		
Coconut	¼ cup (1 oz.)	5.0		
Nature Valley (General Mills):				
Cinnamon & raisin	⅓ cup (1 oz.)	4.0		
Fruit & nut or toasted oat	⅓ cup (1 oz.)	5.0		
NATURE SNACKS (Sun-Maid):				
Carob peanut	1¼ oz.	11.0		
Carob raisin	1¼ oz.	5.0		
Raisin crunch or yogurt crunch	1 oz.	4.3		
Rocky road	1 oz.	4.9		
Yogurt raisin	1 oz.	6.0		
NECTARINE, fresh (USDA) flesh only	4 oz.	Tr.		
NOODLE (USDA):				
Dry, 1½″ strips	1 oz.	1.3	Tr.	1.0
Cooked	1 cup (5.6 oz.)	2.4	< 1.0	2.0
NOODLE & BEEF:				
Canned (Hormel) *Short Orders*	7½-oz. can	14.0		
Frozen (Banquet)	¼ of 32-oz. pkg.	7.0		
NOODLE, CHOW MEIN, CANNED:				
(Chun King)	1 oz.	6.7		
(La Choy)	½ cup (1 oz.)	8.0		
NOODLE MIX:				
*(Betty Crocker):				
Fettucini alfredo	¼ of pkg.	11.0		
Romanoff or stroganoff	¼ of pkg.	12.0		
*(Lipton) & sauce:				
Regular:				
Beef	½ cup	7.0		
Butter, cheese or sour cream & chive	½ cup	9.0		
Deluxe:				
Alfredo or parmesano	½ cup	11.0		
Stroganoff	½ cup	10.0		
NUT, MIXED (See also individual kinds):				
Dry roasted:				
(Planters)	1 oz.	14.2	2.0	12.0
(Skippy)	1 oz.	15.1	2.0	13.0
Oil roasted (Planters):				
With peanuts	1 oz.	14.3		
Without peanuts	1 oz.	15.0		

FOOD DESCRIPTION	MEASURE OR QUANTITY	FATS IN GRAMS		
		Total	Saturated	Unsaturated
NUT & HONEY CRUNCH, cereal (Kellogg's)	⅔ cup (1 oz.)	1.0		
NUTRI-GRAIN, cereal (Kellogg's):				
Almond raisin	⅔ cup (1.4 oz.)	2.0		
Raisin bran	1 cup (1.4 oz.)	1.0		
Wheat	⅔ cup (1 oz.)	0.0		
NUTRIMATO (Mott's)	4 oz.	.3		
OATBAKE, cereal (Kellogg's)	⅓ cup (1 oz.)	3.0		
OAT FLAKES, cereal (Post)	⅔ cup (1 oz.)	1.0		
OATMEAL:				
Instant:				
(H-O):				
Plain	1 T. (4 grams)	.2	Tr.	Tr.
Dates & caramel	1 packet (1.4 oz.)	1.4	Tr.	1.0
Sweet & mellow	1 packet (1.4 oz.)	1.7	Tr.	1.0
*(Quaker):				
Plain 1-oz. packet	¾ cup cooked	1.7		
Apple & cinnamon	1⅛-oz. packet (¾ cup cooked)	1.3		
Chocolate flavor	1¾-oz. packet (¾ cup cooked)	2.0		
Raisins & spice	1½-oz. packet (¾ cup cooked)	1.3		
Quick:				
Dry:				
(H-O)	1 cup (2.5 oz.)	4.1	1.0	3.0
(H-O)	1 T. (4 grams)	.3	Tr.	Tr.
Cooked:				
*(Albers)	1 cup	2.8		
*(Quaker)	⅔ cup (1 oz. dry)	1.7		
Regular:				
Dry:				
(H-O) old-fashioned	1 cup (2.6 oz.)	.4		
(H-O) old-fashioned	1 T. (5 grams)	.3	Tr.	Tr.
*Cooked (Quaker) old-fashioned	⅔ cup (1 oz. dry)	1.7		
OCEAN PERCH (USDA):				
Atlantic:				
Raw, whole	1 lb. (weighed whole)	1.7		
Fried, dipped in egg, milk & bread crumbs	4 oz.	15.1		
Pacific, raw, meat only	4 oz.	1.7		
OCTOPUS, raw, meat only (USDA)	4 oz.	.9		
OIL, salad or cooking:				
Avocado (Calava)	1 T. (.5 oz.)	14.0	2.0	12.0
Canola, *Heart Beat* (GFA)	1 T.	14.0		
Corn:				
(Kraft)	1 oz.	28.4	4.0	24.0
(Mazola)	1 cup (7.7 oz.)	221.0	29.0	192.0
(Mazola)	1 T. (.5 oz.)	14.0	2.0	12.0
Cottonseed (USDA)	½ cup (3.9 oz.)	110.0	28.0	82.0
Olive (USDA)	½ cup (3.9 oz.)	110.0	12.0	98.0
Olive (USDA)	1 T. (.5 oz.)	14.0	2.0	12.0
Peanut (Planter's)	1 T. (.5 oz.)	14.0	3.0	11.0
Safflower:				
(USDA)	½ cup (3.9 oz.)	110.0	9.0	101.0
Saffola	1 T. (.5 oz.)	14.0	1.0	13.0
Sesame (USDA)	½ cup (3.9 oz.)	110.0	15.0	95.0
Soybean (USDA)	1 T. (.5 oz.)	14.0	2.0	12.0
Vegetable, *Crisco* or *Wesson*	1 T.	14.0	3.0	11.0
OKRA:				
Boiled, drained (USDA):				
Whole	½ cup (3.1 oz.)	.3		
Slices	½ cup (2.8 oz.)	.2		
Frozen:				
(Frosty Acres)	3.3 oz.	0.0		
(Ore-Ida) breaded	3 oz.	10.0	2.0	8.0

FOOD DESCRIPTION	MEASURE OR QUANTITY	FATS IN GRAMS		
		Total	Saturated	Unsaturated
OLIVE (USDA):				
Greek-style, salt cured, oil coated:				
Pitted	1 oz.	10.1	1.0	9.0
With pits, drained	4 oz.	32.6	4.0	29.0
Green, pitted & drained	1 oz.	3.6		
Green, pitted & drained	1 olive (13/16″ × 11/16″, 6 grams)	.7		
Ripe, by variety, pitted & drained:				
Ascalano or Manzanilla, any size	1 oz.	3.9	< 1.0	3.0
Mission, any size	1 oz.	5.7	< 1.0	5.0
Mission, slices	½ cup (2.2 oz.)	12.5	1.0	11.0
Sevillano, any size	1 oz.	2.7	Tr.	2.0
ONION:				
Raw (USDA):				
Whole	2½″ onion (3.9 oz.)	.1		
Chopped	½ cup (3 oz.)	< .1		
Grated	1 T. (.5 oz.)	< .1		
Slices	½ cup (2 oz.)	< .1		
Boiled (USDA):				
Whole	½ cup (3.7 oz.)	.1		
Halves or pieces	½ cup (3.2 oz.)	< .1		
Pearl onions	½ cup (3.2 oz.)	< .1		
Canned, boiled, solids & liq. (Comstock-Greenwood)	4 oz.	.1		
Dehydrated (USDA) flakes	1 tsp. (1 gram)	Tr.		
Frozen:				
(Birds Eye):				
Chopped	1 oz.	Tr.		
Pearl, deluxe	⅓ of 10-oz. pkg.	.1		
(Frosty Acres) chopped	1 oz.	0.0		
(Ore-Ida):				
Chopped	2 oz.	< 1.0	< 1.0	< 1.0
Onion Ringers, diced & battered	2 oz.	7.0	1.0	6.0
ONION BOUILLON (Herb-Ox):				
Cube	4-gram cube	.1		
Instant	5-gram packet	.2		
ONION, COCKTAIL (Vlasic) lightly spiced	1 oz.	0.0		
ONION, GREEN, RAW (USDA):				
Whole	1 lb. (weighed untrimmed)	.9		
Slices, bulb & white portion or top	½ cup (1.8 oz.)	.1		
ONION SOUP (See **SOUP,** Onion)				
ONION, WELSH, raw (USDA) trimmed	4 oz.	.5		
OPOSSUM, roasted, meat only (USDA)	4 oz.	11.6		
ORANGE, fresh (USDA):				
All varieties:				
Whole	small orange (2½″ dia., 5.3 oz.)	.2		
Whole	large orange (3⅜″ dia., 8.4 oz.)	.5		
Sections	1 cup (8.5 oz.)	.5		
California Navel:				
Whole	1 lb. (weighed with rind & seeds)	.3		
Sections	1 cup (8.5 oz.)	.2		
California Valencia:				
Fruit, including peel	2⅝″ orange (6.3 oz.)	.5		
Sections	1 cup (8.5 oz.)	.7		
Florida, all varieties:				
Whole	3″-dia. orange (5.5 oz.)	.3		
Sections	1 cup (8.5 oz.)	.5		

FOOD DESCRIPTION	MEASURE OR QUANTITY	FATS IN GRAMS		
		Total	Saturated	Unsaturated
ORANGE DRINK:				
Canned, *Bama* (Borden's)	8.45 fl. oz.	0.0		
*Mix:				
Regular (Funny Face)	6 fl. oz.	0.0		
Dietetic, *Crystal Light*	6 fl. oz.	Tr.		
ORANGE-GRAPEFRUIT JUICE:				
Bottled, chilled (Kraft)	½ cup (4.5 oz.)	.1		
Canned (USDA) sweetened or unsweetened	½ cup (4.4 oz.)	.1		
*Frozen (Minute Maid)	½ cup (4.2 oz.)	Tr.		
ORANGE JUICE:				
Fresh (USDA):				
California Navel	½ cup (4.4 oz.)	.1		
California Valencia	½ cup (4.4 oz.)	.4		
Florida, early or mid-season, temple or Valencia	½ cup (4.4 oz.)	.2		
Chilled, fresh (Citrus Hill)	6 fl. oz.	.2		
Canned or bottled:				
(Borden's) *Sippin' Pak*	8.45 fl. oz.	0.0		
(Johanna Farms) *Tree Ripe*	8.45 fl. oz.	.4		
*Frozen:				
(Birds Eye) *Orange Plus*	6 fl. oz.	.4		
(Citrus Hill)	6 fl. oz.	Tr.		
ORANGE, MANDARIN (See **TANGERINE**)				
ORANGE PEEL (USDA) raw or candied	1 oz.	.1		
ORANGE PINEAPPLE BANANA JUICE, canned (Land O'Lakes)	6 fl. oz.	0.0		
ORANGE PINEAPPLE JUICE, canned (Land O'Lakes)	6 fl. oz.	0.0		
OVEN FRY (General Foods):				
Chicken:				
Extra crispy	4.2-oz. pkg.	8.4		
Homestyle flour	3.2-oz. pkg.	8.2		
Pork, *Shake & Bake*, extra crispy	4.2-oz. pkg.	10.4		
OYSTER (USDA):				
Raw:				
Eastern:				
Meat only	12 oysters (weighed in shell, 4 lbs.)	3.2		
Meat only	19–31 small or 13–19 med. oysters (1 cup, 8.5 oz.)	4.3		
Pacific & Western:				
Meat only	4 oz.	2.5		
Meat only	6–9 small or 4–6 med. oysters (1 cup, 8.5 oz.)	5.3		
Canned, solids & liq.	4 oz.	2.5		
Fried, dipped in egg, milk & bread crumbs	4 oz.	15.8		
Frozen, solids & liq.	4 oz.	6.9		
OYSTER STEW:				
Home recipe (USDA):				
1 part oysters to 1 part milk by volume	1 cup (6–8 oysters, 8.5 oz.)	13.2		
1 part oysters to 3 parts milk by volume	1 cup (8.5 oz.)	12.7		
*Canned (Campbell's)	1 cup	8.0		
*Frozen (USDA):				
Prepared with equal volume water	1 cup (8.5 oz.)	7.7		
Prepared with equal volume milk	1 cup (8.5 oz.)	11.8		
PANCAKE:				
Home recipe (USDA) wheat	4" pancake (1 oz.)	1.8	Tr.	1.0
Frozen (Pillsbury) microwave, any flavor	1 pancake	1.3		

FOOD DESCRIPTION	MEASURE OR QUANTITY	FATS IN GRAMS		
		Total	Saturated	Unsaturated
PANCAKE BATTER, frozen (Aunt Jemima) any flavor	4″ pancake (1.3 oz.)	.5		
PANCAKE DINNER OR ENTREE, frozen (Swanson):				
& blueberry sauce	7-oz. meal	9.0		
& sausage	6-oz. meal	22.0		
& strawberries	7-oz. meal	8.0		
PANCAKE & WAFFLE MIX (See also **PANCAKE & WAFFLE MIX, DIETETIC**):				
*Apple cinnamon, *Bisquick Shake 'N Pour* (General Mills)	4″ pancake	1.7		
*Blueberry:				
Bisquick Shake 'N Pour (General Mills)	4″ pancake	1.7		
FastShake (Little Crow)	½ of 5-oz. container	3.0		
(Pillsbury) *Hungry Jack*	4″ pancake	5.0		
Buttermilk:				
*(Betty Crocker):				
Regular	4″ pancake	3.3		
Complete	4″ pancake	1.0		
FastShake (Little Crow)	½ of 5-oz. container	3.0		
Gold Medal	⅛ of mix	2.0		
*(Mrs. Butterworth's)	4″ pancake	1.0		
*Oat bran, *Bisquick Shake 'N Pour* (General Mills)	4″ pancake	1.3		
*Plain:				
FastShake (Little Crow)	½ of 5-oz. container	4.0		
(Mrs. Butterworth's):				
Regular	4″ pancake	2.0		
Complete	4″ pancake	1.0		
(Pillsbury) *Hungry Jack:*				
Extra Lights:				
Regular	4″ pancake	2.3		
Complete	4″ pancake	.7		
Panshakes	4″ pancake	2.0		
*PANCAKE & WAFFLE MIX, DIETETIC (Estee)	3″ pancake	0.0		
PANCAKE & WAFFLE SYRUP (See **SYRUP,** Pancake & Waffle)				
PANCREAS, raw (USDA):				
Beef, lean only	4 oz.	8.3		
Beef, medium-fat	4 oz.	28.4		
Calf	4 oz.	10.0		
Hog or hog sweetbread	4 oz.	22.6		
PAPAW, fresh (USDA) flesh only	4 oz.	1.0		
PAPAYA, fresh (USDA) flesh only	4 oz.	.1		
PARSLEY, fresh (USDA) chopped	1 T. (4 grams)	Tr.		
PARSNIP (USDA) boiled, drained, cut in pieces	½ cup (3.7 oz.)	.5		
PASSION FRUIT, fresh (USDA) pulp & seeds	4 oz.	.8		
PASTA ACCENTS, frozen (Green Giant):				
Creamy cheddar, garlic or primavera	⅙ of 16-oz. pkg.	5.0	2.0	Tr.
Garden herb	⅙ of 16-oz. pkg.	3.0	Tr.	Tr.
PASTA DINNER OR ENTREE, frozen:				
(Birds Eye):				
Continental style	½ of 10-oz. pkg.	8.0		
Primavera, For One	5-oz. pkg.	9.5		
(Celentano) & cheese, baked	½ of 12-oz. pkg.	7.0		
(Green Giant):				
Dijon	9½-oz. pkg.	17.0	9.0	1.0
Marinara, one serving	6-oz. pkg.	5.0	Tr.	1.0

FOOD DESCRIPTION	MEASURE OR QUANTITY	FATS IN GRAMS		
		Total	Saturated	Unsaturated
Parmesan, with sweet peas, one serving	5½-oz. pkg.	5.0	2.0	0.0
(Stouffer's):				
Carbonara	9¾-oz. pkg.	45.0		
Mexicali	10-oz. pkg.	31.0		
Primavera	10⅝-oz. pkg.	21.0		
(Weight Watchers):				
Primavera	8½-oz. pkg.	11.0	Tr.	11.0
Rigati	11-oz. pkg.	9.0	3.0	6.0
PASTA SALAD, frozen (Birds Eye) classic, Italian-style	½ of 10-oz. pkg.	7.0		
ʼPASTA & SAUCE, mix (Lipton):				
Cheddar broccoli with fusilli	¼ of pkg.	1.8		
Cheese supreme	¼ of pkg.	2.3		
Garlic, creamy	¼ of pkg.	.8		
Mushroom & chicken	¼ of pkg.	2.6		
PASTINAS, dry (USDA):				
Carrot or spinach	1 oz.	.5		
Egg	1 oz.	1.2	Tr.	Tr.
PASTRAMI, packaged:				
(Carl Buddig)	1 oz.	2.0	.9	1.0
Hebrew National	1 oz.	1.4		
(Oscar Mayer)	.6-oz. slice	.3	.2	.2
PASTRY SHEET, PUFF, frozen (Pepperidge Farm)	1 sheet	68.0		
PASTRY SHELL (See also **PIE CRUST**):				
Home recipe (USDA):				
Made with lard, baked	1 shell (1.5 oz.)	14.2	6.0	9.0
Made with vegetable shortening, baked	1 shell (1.5 oz.)	14.2	3.0	11.0
Frozen (Pet-Ritz)	3″ shell	10.0		
PÂTÉ, canned:				
De foie gras (USDA)	1 oz.	12.4		
Liver (Hormel)	1 T.	3.0		
PEA, GREEN:				
Raw (USDA):				
Shelled	1 lb.	1.8		
Shelled	½ cup (2.4 oz.)	.3		
Boiled, drained (USDA)	½ cup (2.9 oz.)	.3		
Canned, regular pack, solids & liq.:				
(Green Giant):				
Early June, with onions	¼ of 17-oz. can	.2		
Sweet	½ of 8.5-oz. can	.4		
(Le Sueur) early	½ of 8.5-oz. can	.2		
Canned, dietetic pack, solids & liq.:				
(Diet Delight)	½ cup (4.4 oz.)	.2		
(S & W) *Nutradiet,* unseasoned	4 oz.	.1		
Frozen:				
(Birds Eye):				
In cream sauce	⅓ of pkg (2.7 oz.)	7.0		
Tender, tiny	3.3 oz.	.3		
(Green Giant):				
In butter sauce	½ cup	1.0		
With cream sauce	½ cup	4.0		
PEA, MATURE SEED, dry (USDA):				
Raw:				
Whole	1 cup (7.1 oz.)	2.6		
Split, without seed coat	1 lb.	4.5		
Split, without seed coat	1 cup (7.2 oz.)	2.0		
Cooked, split, without seed coat, drained	½ cup (3.4 oz.)	.3		
PEA & CARROT:				
Canned, regular pack, solids & liq., (Comstock)	½ cup (4.4 oz.)	0.0		

FOOD DESCRIPTION	MEASURE OR QUANTITY	FATS IN GRAMS		
		Total	Saturated	Unsaturated
Canned, dietetic pack, solids & liq. (Diet Delight)	1/2 cup (4.2 oz.)	0.0		
Frozen:				
(Birds Eye)	1/2 cup (3.3 oz.)	.4		
(Frosty Acres)	3.3 oz.	0.0		
PEA & ONION, frozen (Larsen)	3.3 oz.	0.0		
PEA POD, edible-podded or Chinese (USDA):				
Raw	1 lb. (weighed untrimmed)	.9		
Boiled, drained	4 oz.	.2		
PEACH:				
Fresh, without skin (USDA):				
Whole	4-oz. peach (2 1/2" dia.)	.1		
Diced or slices	1/2 cup	.1		
Canned, regular pack, solids & liq.:				
(USDA):				
Juice pack, light syrup or extra heavy syrup	4 oz.	.1		
Heavy syrup, halves	1/2 cup (4.5 oz.)	.1		
(Hunt's) heavy syrup, diced	5 oz.	Tr.		
Canned, dietetic or unsweetened, solids & liq.:				
(USDA) water pack	1/2 cup (4.3 oz.)	.1		
(Del Monte) lite, cling	1/2 cup (4 oz.)	0.0		
Dehydrated, sulfured, nugget or pieces (USDA):				
Uncooked	1 oz.	.3		
Cooked with added sugar, solids & liq.	1/2 cup (5–6 halves & 3 T. liq., 5.4 oz.)	.3		
Dried (USDA):				
Uncooked	1/2 cup (3.1 oz.)	.6		
Cooked, unsweetened	1/2 cup (5–6 halves & 3 T. liq., 4.8 oz.)	.3		
Frozen (Birds Eye) quick thaw	1/2 cup (5 oz.)	.2		
PEACH BUTTER (Smucker's)	1 T. (.6 oz.)	Tr.		
PEACH JUICE, canned (Smucker's)	8 fl. oz.	0.0		
PEACH NECTAR, canned (Libby's)	1 cup (8.7 oz.)	0.0		
PEACH PRESERVE:				
Sweetened (Bama)	1 T.	0.0		
Dietetic (Featherweight)	1 T.	0.0		
PEANUT:				
Raw (USDA):				
In shell	1 lb. (weighed in shell)	157.3	35.0	122.0
With or without skins, whole	1 oz.	13.7	3.0	11.0
Boiled (USDA)	1 oz.	8.9	2.0	7.0
Roasted:				
(USDA):				
With skins, unsalted	1 oz.	13.5	3.0	11.0
Without skins, salted	1 oz.	14.1	3.0	11.0
Halves, salted	1/2 cup (2.5 oz.)	35.9	8.0	38.0
Chopped, salted	1 T. (9 grams)	4.5	1.0	3.0
(Eagle):				
Fancy Virginia	1 oz.	16.0		
Honey Roast, regular, cinnamon or maple	1 oz.	13.0		
Lightly salted	1 oz.	15.0		
(Planters):				
In shell, salted or unsalted	1 oz.	14.0		
Dry roasted:				
Salted	1 oz.	14.0		
Unsalted	1 oz.	15.0		

FOOD DESCRIPTION	MEASURE OR QUANTITY	FATS IN GRAMS		
		Total	Saturated	Unsaturated
Oil roasted:				
Salted, tavern nuts or unsalted	1 oz.	15.0		
Sweet & crunchy	1 oz.	8.0		
(Weight Watchers)	1 pouch	7.0		
PEANUT BUTTER:				
(Algood) crunchy, old-fashioned or smooth	1 T.	8.0	1.5	2.5
Jif, creamy or extra crunchy	1 T.	7.8	1.1	6.2
(Peter Pan) creamy, crunchy or low-sodium	1 T.	8.0		
(Skippy):				
Creamy	1 T.	8.2	1.7	6.4
Super chunk	1 T.	8.4	1.7	6.6
(Smucker's) natural or honey sweetened	1 T.	8.0	1.5	6.5
PEANUT BUTTER MORSELS:				
(Nestlé's)	1 oz.	10.0		
(Reese's)	1 oz.	8.7		
PEAR:				
Fresh (USDA):				
Whole	6.4-oz. pear (3″ × 2½″)	.6		
Quartered	½ cup (3.4 oz.)	.4		
Canned, regular pack, solids & liq.:				
(USDA):				
Juice pack	4 oz.	.3		
Light syrup, heavy syrup or extra heavy syrup	1 oz.	.2		
(Del Monte) heavy syrup	½ cup (4 oz.)	.6		
(Stokely-Van Camp's)	½ cup (4 oz.)	.2		
Canned, unsweetened or low-calorie, solids & liq.:				
(USDA) water pack	½ cup (4.3 oz.)	.2		
(Diet Delight) halves or quarters	½ cup (4.4 oz.)	Tr.		
Dried:				
(USDA) cooked, with or without added sugar, solids & liq.	4 oz.	.9		
(Del Monte) uncooked	½ cup (2.8 oz.)	.6		
PEAR NECTAR, sweetened (USDA)	1 cup (8.5 oz.)	.5		
PEBBLES, cereal (Post) cocoa or fruity	⅞ cup (1 oz.)	1.0		
PECAN:				
In shell (USDA)	1 lb. (weighed in shell)	171.2	12.0	159.0
Shelled (USDA) unsalted:				
Whole	1 lb.	323.0	23.0	300.0
Halves	12–14 halves (.5 oz.)	10.0	Tr.	9.0
Chopped	1 T. (7 grams)	5.0	Tr.	5.0
Roasted, dry (Fisher)	1 oz.	18.0		
PECTIN, FRUIT:				
Certo	6-oz. pkg.	0.0		
Sure-Jell, regular or light	1¾-oz. pkg.	0.0		
PEPPER:				
Black:				
(USDA)	1 tsp. (2 grams)	.2		
Seasoned (Lawry's)	1 tsp. (2 grams)	.1		
Lemon (Durkee)	1 tsp.	Tr.		
PEPPER, BANANA (Vlasic) hot rings	1 oz.	0.0		
PEPPER, CHERRY (Vlasic) mild	1 oz.	0.0		
PEPPER, HOT CHILI:				
Green (USDA):				
Raw, whole or without seeds	4 oz.	.2		
Canned, pods, without seeds, solids & liq.	4 oz.	1.1		

FOOD DESCRIPTION	MEASURE OR QUANTITY	FATS IN GRAMS		
		Total	Saturated	Unsaturated
Red:				
Raw, whole (USDA)	4 oz. (weighed with seeds)	2.6		
Raw, trimmed, pods only (USDA)	4 oz.	3.2		
Canned:				
(Del Monte) solids & liq.	¼ cup	.3		
(Ortega) drained	¼ cup (1.8 oz.)	.1		
Dried (USDA) pods	1 oz.	2.6		
PEPPER, STUFFED:				
Home recipe, with beef & crumbs (USDA)	2¾" × 2½" pepper with 1⅛ cups stuffing (6.5 oz.)	10.2	6.0	5.0
Frozen (Stouffer's)	½ of 15½-oz. pkg.	9.0		
PEPPER, SWEET:				
Green:				
Raw (USDA):				
Whole	1 lb. (weighed untrimmed)	.7		
Without stem & seeds	1 med. pepper (2.6 oz.)	.1		
Chopped	½ cup (2.6 oz.)	.2		
Boiled (USDA) drained	1 med. pepper (2.6 oz.)	.1		
Frozen (Larsen)	1 oz.	0.0		
Red:				
Raw (USDA):				
Whole	1 lb. (weighed with stems & seeds)	1.1		
Without stem & seeds	1 med. pepper (2.2 oz.)	.2		
Frozen (Larsen)	1 oz.	0.0		
PEPPERONCINI (Vlasic) Greek, mild	1 oz.	0.0		
PEPPERONI:				
(Eckrich)	1 oz.	12.0		
(Hormel):				
Regular, *Rosa* or *Rosa Grande*	1 oz.	13.0		
Canned, bits	1 T.	3.0		
Sliced, packaged	1 slice	3.5		
PEPPER STEAK:				
*Canned:				
(Chun King) stir fry	6-oz. serving	16.6		
(La Choy)	¾ cup	9.0		
Frozen:				
(Armour):				
Classics Lite	11¼-oz. pkg.	4.0		
Dining Lite	9-oz. pkg.	6.0		
(Healthy Choice) beef:				
Dinner	11-oz. dinner	6.0	3.0	Tr.
Entree	9½-oz. entree	4.0	2.0	Tr.
(Stouffer's)	10½-oz. meal	11.0		
PERCH:				
Raw (USDA):				
White, meat only	4 oz.	4.5		
Yellow, meat only	4 oz.	1.0		
Frozen:				
(Gorton's) *Fishmarket Fresh*	4-oz. fillet	3.0		
(Van de Kamp's):				
Regular, batter dipped	2-oz. piece	7.5		
Today's Catch	4 oz.	0.0		
PERSIMMON (USDA):				
Japanese or Kaki, fresh:				
With seeds or seedless	1 lb. (weighed with skin, calyx & seeds)	1.5		
With seeds or seedless	4.4-oz. persimmon	.4		
Native, fresh, flesh only	4 oz.	.5		
PHEASANT, raw (USDA):				
Meat & skin	4 oz.	5.9		
Meat only	4 oz.	7.7		
Giblets	2 oz.	2.8		
PICKEREL, chain, raw (USDA)				
meat only	4 oz.	.6		

FOOD DESCRIPTION	MEASURE OR QUANTITY	FATS IN GRAMS		
		Total	Saturated	Unsaturated
PICKLE:				
Chow chow (See **CHOW CHOW**)				
Cucumber, fresh or bread & butter:				
(Fanning's)	1 fl. oz.	Tr.		
(Vlasic) chips, chunks or stix	1 oz.	0.0		
Dill:				
(Heinz)	3" pickle	.1		
(Vlasic) original or no garlic	1 oz.	0.0		
Hamburger (Vlasic) dill, chips	1 oz.	0.0		
Kosher dill:				
(Claussen) whole	1.9-oz. pickle	.1		
(Vlasic) baby, crunchy, dill or spears	1 oz.	0.0		
Sour, cucumber (USDA)	1¾" × 4" pickle (4.8 oz.)	.3		
Sweet, cucumber (USDA):				
Whole, gherkin	2½" × ¾" pickle (.5 oz.)	Tr.		
Chopped	½ cup (2.6 oz.)	.3		
PIE:				
Regular, non-frozen:				
Apple:				
Home recipe (USDA) 2-crust	⅙ of 9" pie	17.5	6.3	11.2
(Dolly Madison)	4½-oz. pie	27.0		
Banana, home recipe (USDA) cream or custard	⅙ of 9" pie	14.1		
Blackberry, home recipe (USDA):				
2-crust, made with lard	⅙ of 9" pie (5.6 oz.)	17.4	6.0	11.0
2-crust, made with vegetable shortening	⅙ of 9" pie (5.6 oz.)	17.4	5.0	13.0
Blueberry:				
Home recipe (USDA) 2-crust	⅙ of 9" pie	17.1	6.3	10.7
(Dolly Madison)	4½-oz. pie	21.0		
Boston cream (USDA) home recipe	1/12 of 8" pie	6.5		
Cherry:				
Home recipe (USDA) 2-crust	⅙ of 9" pie	17.9	6.3	11.5
(Dolly Madison):				
Regular	4½-oz. pie	27.0		
& cream	4½-oz. pie	19.0		
Chocolate (Dolly Madison):				
Regular	4½-oz. pie	28.0		
Pudding	4½-oz. pie	30.0		
Chocolate meringue (USDA) home recipe	⅙ of 9" pie	16.8	5.6	11.2
Coconut custard (USDA) home recipe	⅙ of 9" pie	19.0		
Lemon (Dolly Madison)	4½-oz. pie	23.0		
Lemon meringue (USDA) home recipe, 1-crust	⅙ of 9" pie	14.3	5.2	9.1
Mince (USDA) home recipe, 2-crust	⅙ of 9" pie	18.2		
Peach (Dolly Madison)	4½-oz. pie	26.0		
Pumpkin (USDA) home recipe, 1-crust	⅙ of 9" pie	17.0	6.1	10.9
Strawberry (Dolly Madison)	4½-oz. pie	19.0		
Frozen:				
Apple:				
(Banquet) family size	⅙ of 20-oz. pie	11.0		
(Mrs. Smith's):				
Regular:				
Plain	⅛ of 10" pie (5¾ oz.)	18.0	3.0	15.0
Dutch	⅛ of 8" pie (3¼ oz.)	11.0	2.0	9.0

FOOD DESCRIPTION	MEASURE OR QUANTITY	FATS IN GRAMS		
		Total	Saturated	Unsaturated
Natural Juice:				
Plain	⅛ of 9" pie (4.6 oz.)	20.0	4.0	16.0
Dutch	⅛ of 9" pie (5.12 oz.)	16.0	3.0	13.0
Pie in Minutes	⅛ of pie (3.1 oz.)	9.0	2.0	7.0
(Pet-Ritz)	⅙ of 26-oz. pie	12.0		
(Weight Watchers)	3½ oz.	5.0	1.0	4.0
Banana cream:				
(Banquet)	⅙ of 14-oz. pie	10.0		
(Pet-Ritz)	⅙ of 14-oz. pie	9.0		
Blueberry:				
(Mrs. Smith's):				
Regular	⅛ of 8" pie (3¼ oz.)	10.0	2.0	8.0
Pie in Minutes	⅛ of pie (3.1 oz.)	9.0	2.0	7.0
(Pet-Ritz)	⅙ of 26-oz. pie	12.0		
Cherry:				
(Banquet)	⅙ of 20-oz. pie	11.0		
(Mrs. Smith's):				
Natural Juice	⅛ of 36.8-oz. pie	16.0	3.0	13.0
Pie in Minutes	⅛ of 25-oz. pie	9.0	2.0	7.0
(Pet-Ritz)	⅙ of 26-oz. pie	12.0		
Chocolate cream:				
(Banquet)	⅙ of 14-oz. pie	10.0		
(Pet-Ritz)	⅙ of 14-oz. pie	8.0		
Chocolate mocha (Weight Watchers)	2¾-oz. serving	5.0	3.0	<3.0
Coconut cream (Banquet)	⅙ of 14-oz. pie	11.0		
Coconut custard (Mrs. Smith's):				
8" pie	⅛ of 25-oz. pie	9.0	4.0	5.0
10" pie	⅛ of 44-oz. pie	12.0	3.0	9.0
Custard, egg (Pet-Ritz)	⅙ of 24-oz. pie	8.0		
Lemon cream:				
(Banquet)	⅙ of 14-oz. pie	9.0		
(Pet-Ritz)	⅙ of 14-oz. pie	9.0		
Lemon meringue (Mrs. Smith's)	⅛ of 8" pie (3 oz.)	5.0	1.0	4.0
Mincemeat:				
(Banquet) family size	⅙ of 20-oz. pie	11.0		
(Mrs. Smith's):				
26-oz. pie	⅛ of pie (3¼ oz.)	11.0	2.0	9.0
46-oz. pie	⅛ of pie (5¾ oz.)	18.0	3.0	15.0
Peach:				
(Banquet) family size	⅙ of 20-oz. pie	11.0		
(Mrs. Smith's):				
Regular	⅛ of 26-oz. pie	10.0	2.0	8.0
Natural Juice	⅛ of 36.8-oz. pie	15.0	3.0	12.0
Pie in Minutes	⅛ of 25-oz. pie	9.0	2.0	7.0
(Pet-Ritz)	⅙ of 26-oz. pie	12.0		
Pecan (Mrs. Smith's):				
Regular	⅛ of 24-oz. pie	13.0	2.0	11.0
Pie in Minutes	⅛ of 24-oz. pie	13.0	2.0	11.0
Pumpkin:				
(Banquet)	⅙ of 20-oz. pie	8.0		
(Mrs. Smith's) *Pie in Minutes*	⅛ of 25-oz. pie	6.0	2.0	4.0
Pumpkin custard:				
(Mrs. Smith's)	⅛ of 46-oz. pie	10.0	2.0	8.0
(Pet-Ritz)	⅙ of 26-oz. pie	9.0		
Strawberry cream:				
(Banquet)	⅙ of 14-oz. pie	9.0		
(Pet-Ritz)	⅙ of 14-oz. pie	9.0		
Sweet potato (Pet-Ritz)	⅙ of 20-oz. pie	7.0		
PIECRUST (See also **PASTRY SHELL**):				
Home recipe (USDA) baked, 9" crust:				
Made with lard	1 crust (6.3 oz.)	60.1	23.0	37.0
Made with vegetable shortening	1 crust (6.3 oz.)	60.1	14.0	46.0

FOOD DESCRIPTION	MEASURE OR QUANTITY	Total	Saturated	Unsaturated
Frozen:				
(Empire Kosher)	7-oz. pkg.	63.0		
(Mrs. Smith's):				
8" or 9" pie shell	1/8 of shell	5.0	1.0	4.0
95/8" shell	1/8 of 15-oz. shell	7.0	1.0	4.0
(Oronoque) deep dish	1/6 of 8½-oz. shell	13.0		
(Pet-Ritz):				
Regular	1/6 of 5-oz. pkg.	7.0		
Deep dish:				
Regular	1/6 of 6-oz. pkg.	8.0		
All vegetable shortening	1/6 of 6-oz. pkg.	9.0		
Graham cracker	1/6 of 5-oz. pkg.	6.0		
PIECRUST MIX:				
(USDA):				
Dry, pkg. or stick	10-oz. pkg. (2 crusts)	92.9	20.0	73.0
*Prepared with water, baked	4 oz.	33.0	8.0	25.0
(Betty Crocker)	1/6 of pkg. or 1/8 of stick	8.0		
*(Flako)	1/6 of 9" piecrust	14.5		
*(Pillsbury) mix or stick	1/6 of 2-crust pie shell	17.0		
PIE FILLING (See also **PUDDING OR PIE FILLING**):				
Apple:				
(Comstock)	1/6 of 21-oz. can	1.0		
(White House)	1/2 cup (4.8 oz.)	1.0		
Apple rings or slices (See **APPLE,** canned)				
Banana cream (Comstock)	1/6 of 21-oz. can	4.0		
Blackberry:				
(Comstock)	1 cup (10¾ oz.)	Tr.		
(Lucky Leaf)	8 oz.	.4		
Blueberry (White House)	1/2 cup	1.0		
Cherry (Thank You Brand) regular	3½ oz.	0.0		
Coconut cream (Comstock)	1/6 of 21-oz. can	4.0		
Lemon (Comstock)	1/6 of 21-oz. can	4.0		
Mincemeat (Comstock)	1/2 of 21-oz. can	4.0		
Peach (White House)	1/2 cup (4.8 oz.)	1.0		
Pumpkin (Libby's) (See also **PUMPKIN,** canned)	1 cup	0.0		
Raisin (Comstock)	1/6 of 21-oz. can	2.0		
*PIE MIX:				
Boston cream (Betty Crocker)	1/8 of pie	6.0		
Chocolate (Royal) No Bake	1/8 of pie	15.0		
PIEROGIE, frozen (Empire Kosher):				
Cheese	1½ oz.	5.0		
Onion	1½ oz.	4.0		
PIGEON (See **SQUAB**)				
PIGEONPEA (USDA):				
Raw, immature seeds in pods	1 lb.	1.1		
Dry seeds	1 lb.	6.4		
PIGS FEET, pickled (USDA)	4 oz.	16.8	6.0	11.0
PIKE, raw (USDA):				
Blue, meat only	4 oz.	1.0		
Northern, meat only	4 oz.	1.2		
Walleye, meat only	4 oz.	1.4		
PILI NUT (USDA) shelled	4 oz.	80.6		
PIMIENTO, canned:				
(Dromedary) whole pods, slices, pieces	1 oz.	0.0		
(Sunshine) diced or sliced, solids & liq.	1 T. (.6 oz.)	Tr.		
PINA COLADA, mix:				
*(Bar-Tender's)	5 fl. oz.	3.0		
(Holland House):				
Liquid	1 oz.	0.0		
Instant	.5 oz.	3.0		

FOOD DESCRIPTION	MEASURE OR QUANTITY	FATS IN GRAMS		
		Total	Saturated	Unsaturated
PINEAPPLE:				
Fresh (USDA):				
Whole	1 lb. (weighed untrimmed)	.5		
Diced	1/2 cup (2.8 oz.)	.2		
Slices	3/4" × 31/2" slice (3 oz.)	.2		
Canned, regular pack, solids & liq.:				
(USDA):				
Juice pack, light syrup or water pack	4 oz.	.1		
Heavy syrup:				
Crushed	1/2 cup (4.6 oz.)	.1		
Slices	1/2 cup (4.9 oz.)	.1		
(Del Monte):				
Juice pack	1/2 cup (4.9 oz.)	.3		
Heavy syrup	1/2 cup (5 oz.)	0.0		
(Dole):				
Juice pack:				
Chunks or crushed	1/2 cup (includes 21/2 T. juice, 3.7 oz.)	.1		
Slices	2 med. slices & 21/2 T. juice (3.7 oz.)	.1		
Heavy syrup, chunks, crushed, tidbits or slices	4 oz.	.1		
Frozen:				
(USDA) chunks, sweetened, not thawed	1/2 cup (4.3 oz.)	.1		
(Dole) chunks in heavy syrup	11 chunks & 21/2 T. syrup (4 oz.)	.1		
PINEAPPLE, CANDIED				
(USDA)	1 oz.	.1		
PINEAPPLE & GRAPEFRUIT JUICE DRINK, canned:				
(USDA) 40% fruit juices	1/2 cup (4.4 oz.)	Tr.		
(Del Monte)	1/2 cup (4.3 oz.)	0.0		
PINEAPPLE JUICE:				
Canned, unsweetened:				
(Del Monte)	1/2 cup (4.3 oz.)	0.0		
(Dole)	6-fl.-oz. can	.2		
*Frozen, unsweetened (Minute Maid)	6 fl. oz.	.2		
PINEAPPLE & ORANGE JUICE DRINK, canned:				
(USDA) 40% fruit juices	1/2 cup (4.4 oz.)	.1		
(Johanna Farms) *Tree-Ripe*	8.45-fl.-oz. container	.1		
PINEAPPLE PRESERVE:				
Sweetened (Home Brand)	1 T. (.7 oz.)	0.0		
Low-calorie (Tillie Lewis)	1 T. (.5 oz.)	Tr.		
PINE NUT (USDA):				
Pignolias, shelled	4 oz.	53.8		
Pinon, shelled	4 oz.	68.6		
PISTACHIO NUT:				
(USDA):				
In shell	4 oz. (weighed in shell)	30.4	3.0	27.0
Shelled	1/2 cup (2.2 oz.)	33.3	3.0	30.0
(Planters) in shell, red or natural, salted	1 oz.	15.0		
PITANGA, fresh (USDA) flesh only	4 oz.	.5		
PIZZA PIE (See also **SHAKEY'S**):				
Home recipe, with cheese topping:				
(USDA)	4 oz.	9.4	3.0	6.0
(USDA)	51/2" sector (1/8 of 14" pie, 2.5 oz.)	6.2	2.0	4.0

FOOD DESCRIPTION	MEASURE OR QUANTITY	Total	Saturated	Unsaturated
Home recipe, with sausage topping:				
(USDA)	4 oz.	10.5	3.0	7.0
(USDA)	5½" sector (⅛ of 14" pie, 2.6 oz.)	7.0	2.0	5.0
Chilled, baked (USDA)	4 oz.	7.7	2.0	5.0
Regular, non-frozen:				
Domino's:				
Cheese:				
Plain:				
12" pizza	1 slice	4.2		
16" pizza	1 slice	5.1		
Double cheese:				
12" pizza	1 slice	7.8		
16" pizza	1 slice	9.4		
Double, with pepperoni:				
12" pizza	1 slice	11.1		
16" pizza	1 slice	13.0		
Mushroom & sausage:				
12" pizza	1 slice	6.3		
16" pizza	1 slice	7.3		
Pepperoni:				
Plain:				
12" pizza	1 slice	7.5		
16" pizza	1 slice	8.7		
Mushroom:				
12" pizza	1 slice	7.5		
16" pizza	1 slice	8.5		
Sausage:				
12" pizza	1 slice	9.5		
16" pizza	1 slice	10.0		
Sausage:				
12" pizza	1 slice	6.3		
16" pizza	1 slice	7.3		
Godfather's:				
Cheese:				
Original:				
Small	⅙ of pie (3.6 oz.)	7.0		
Medium	⅛ of pie (4 oz.)	8.0		
Large:				
Regular	1/10 of pie (4.4 oz.)	9.0		
Hot slice	⅛ of pie (5.5 oz.)	11.0		
Stuffed:				
Small	1/16 of pie (4.4 oz.)	11.0		
Large	1/10 of pie (5.2 oz.)	16.0		
Thin crust:				
Medium	⅛ of pie (3 oz.)	7.0		
Large	1/10 of pie (3.4 oz.)	7.0		
Combo:				
Original:				
Small	⅙ of pie (5.6 oz.)	15.0		
Medium	⅛ of pie (6.2 oz.)	17.0		
Large:				
Regular	1/10 of pie (6.8 oz.)	19.0		
Hot slice	⅛ of pie (8.5 oz.)	24.0		
Stuffed:				
Small	⅙ of pie (6.3 oz.)	20.0		
Large	1/10 of pie (7.6 oz.)	26.0		
Thin crust:				
Medium	⅛ of pie (4.9 oz.)	14.0		
Large	1/10 of pie (5.4 oz.)	16.0		
Frozen:				
Bacon (Totino's)	½ of 10-oz. pie	20.0		
Bagel (Empire Kosher)	2-oz. serving	4.0		
Canadian-style bacon:				
(Jeno's) Crisp'n Tasty	½ of 7.7-oz. pie	11.0		
(Stouffer's) french bread	½ of 11⅝-oz. pkg.	14.0		
Cheese:				
(Banquet) Zap, french bread	4½-oz. serving	10.0		

FOOD DESCRIPTION	MEASURE OR QUANTITY	FATS IN GRAMS		
		Total	Saturated	Unsaturated
(Celentano):				
Mini slice	2.7-oz. slice	4.0		
Thick crust	1/3 of 13-oz. pie	11.0		
(Empire Kosher):				
Family size	1/5 of 15-oz. pie	7.0		
3-pack	1/9 of 27-oz. pkg.	7.0		
(Jeno's):				
Crisp'n Tasty	1/2 of 7.4-oz. pie	14.0		
4-pack	1/4 of 8.9-oz. pkg.	8.0		
(Kid Cuisine)	6 1/2-oz. serving	4.0		
(Pappalo's) french bread	5.7-oz. serving	15.0		
(Pillsbury):				
Regular	1/2 of 7.1-oz. pie	10.0		
French bread	5.7-oz. serving	15.0		
(Stouffer's) french bread:				
Regular:				
Plain	1/2 of 10 3/8-oz. pkg.	13.0		
Double cheese	1/2 of 11 3/4-oz. pkg.	18.0		
Lean Cuisine:				
Regular	5 1/2-oz. serving	10.0		
Extra cheese	5 1/2-oz. serving	12.0		
(Totino's):				
Microwave, small	3.9-oz. serving	8.0		
Pan, three cheese	1/6 of 23.4-oz. pie	10.0		
Slices	2 1/2-oz. piece	7.0		
(Weight Watchers):				
Regular	5 3/4-oz. serving	8.0	2.0	6.0
French bread	5.1-oz. serving	12.0	5.0	7.0
Combination:				
(Jeno's):				
Crisp'n Tasty	1/2 of 7.8-oz. pie	16.0		
4-pack	1/4 of 9.6-oz. pkg.	9.0		
(Pappalo's):				
French bread	6 1/2-oz. serving	21.0		
Pan	1/6 of 26 1/2-oz. pie	15.0		
(Pillsbury) microwave	1/2 of 9-oz. pie	15.0		
(Totino's):				
My Classic, deluxe	1/6 of 22 1/2-oz. pie	12.0		
Slices	2.7-oz. slice	10.0		
(Weight Watchers) deluxe	6 3/4-oz. serving	8.0	1.0	7.0
Deluxe:				
(Banquet) Zap, french bread	4.8-oz. serving	13.0		
(Stouffer's) french bread:				
Regular	1/2 of 12 3/8-oz. pkg.	21.0		
Lean Cuisine	6 1/8-oz. serving	12.0		
(Weight Watchers) french bread	6.12-oz. serving	13.0	3.0	10.0
English muffin (Empire Kosher)	2-oz. serving	4.0		
Hamburger:				
(Fox Deluxe)	1/2 of 7.6-oz. pie	12.0		
(Pappalo's):				
Pan	1/6 of 26.3-oz. pie	12.0		
Thin crust	1/6 of 22-oz. pie	8.0		
(Stouffer's) french bread	1/2 of 12 1/4-oz. pkg.	19.0		
(Totino's) party	1/2 of 10.6-oz. pkg.	19.0		
Mexican-style (Totino's)	1/2 of 10.2-oz. pkg.	21.0		
Pepperoni:				
(Fox Deluxe)	1/2 of 7-oz. pie	13.0		
(Jeno's) Crisp'n Tasty	1/2 of 7.6-oz. pie	15.0		
(Pappalo's):				
French bread	6-oz. piece	20.0		
Thin crust	1/6 of 22-oz. pie	11.0		
(Pillsbury) microwave:				
Regular	1/2 of 8 1/2-oz. pie	15.0		
French bread	6-oz. piece	19.0		
(Stouffer's) french bread:				
Regular	1/2 of 11 1/4-oz. pie	20.0		
Lean Cuisine	5 1/2-oz. piece	12.0		

FOOD DESCRIPTION	MEASURE OR QUANTITY	FATS IN GRAMS		
		Total	Saturated	Unsaturated
(Totino's):				
Microwave, small	4-oz. pie	12.0		
My Classic	⅙ of 21.1-oz. pie	13.0		
Party	½ of 10.2-oz. pie	20.0		
(Weight Watchers):				
Regular	5.87-oz. serving	9.0	3.0	6.0
French bread	5¼-oz. serving	14.0	5.0	8.0
Pepperoni & Mushroom				
(Stouffer's) french bread	½ of 12¼-oz. pkg.	22.0		
Sausage:				
(Fox Deluxe)	½ of 7.2-oz. pie	13.0		
(Jeno's) Crisp'n Tasty	½ of 7.8-oz. pie	16.0		
(Pappalo's) french bread	9.6-oz. piece	18.0		
(Pillsbury) microwave:				
Regular	½ of 8¾-oz. pkg.	13.0		
French bread	6.3-oz. serving	16.0		
(Stouffer's) french bread:				
Regular	½ of 12-oz. pkg.	20.0		
Lean Cuisine	6-oz. serving	11.0		
(Totino's):				
Microwave, small	4-oz. pie	16.0		
Party	½ of 10.6-oz. pie	21.0		
Slices	2.7-oz. piece	10.0		
(Weight Watchers)	6¼-oz. serving	8.0	2.0	6.0
Sausage & mushroom				
(Stouffer's) french bread	½ of 12½-oz. pkg.	19.0		
Sausage & pepperoni:				
(Fox Deluxe)	½ of 7.2-oz. pie	13.0		
(Stouffer's) french bread	½ of 12½-oz. pkg.	23.0		
(Totino's) pan	⅙ of 26.6-oz. pie	15.0		
Vegetable:				
(Stouffer's) french bread	½ of 12¾-oz. pie	20.0		
(Totino's) party	½ of 10.7-oz. pie	13.0		
PIZZA PIE CRUST:				
*Mix, *Gold Medal*	⅙ of mix	1.0		
Refrigerated (Pillsbury) all ready	⅛ of crust	1.0	Tr.	Tr.
PIZZA ROLL, frozen (Jeno's):				
Cheese	3 oz.	12.0		
Hamburger, pepperoni & cheese or sausage & pepperoni	3 oz.	13.0		
PIZZA SAUCE, canned:				
(Contadina):				
Regular, with cheese or pepperoni	½ cup	4.0		
With tomato chunks	½ cup	0.0		
(Ragú) *Pizza Quick:*				
Chunky	4 oz.	4.1		
Pepperoni	4 oz.	7.1		
PLANTAIN, raw (USDA) flesh only	4 oz.	.5		
PLUM:				
Fresh (USDA):				
Damson, flesh only	4 oz.	Tr.		
Japanese & hybrid:				
Whole	2″ plum (2.1 oz.)	.1		
Diced, halves or slices	½ cup	.2		
Prune-type, fresh (USDA):				
Whole	1 lb. (weighed with pits)	.9		
Halves	½ cup (2.8 oz.)	.2		
Canned, purple, regular pack, solids & liq.:				
(USDA):				
Light syrup	4 oz.	.1		
Heavy syrup, with or without pits	½ cup	.1		
(Del Monte) heavy syrup	½ cup (4.1 oz.)	.1		

FOOD DESCRIPTION	MEASURE OR QUANTITY	FATS IN GRAMS		
		Total	Saturated	Unsaturated
Canned, unsweetened or low-calorie, solids & liq.:				
Greengage, water pack (USDA)	4 oz.	.1		
Purple:				
(USDA) water pack	4 oz.	.2		
(Diet Delight)	½ cup (4.4 oz.)	Tr.		
PLUM PRESERVE OR JAM, sweetened, Damson or red (Bama)	1 T. (.7 oz.)	0.0		
PLUM PUDDING (Richardson & Robbins)	2" piece (3.6 oz.)	1.0		
POLLOCK (USDA):				
Raw, meat only	4 oz.	1.0		
Creamed, prepared with flour, butter & milk	4 oz.	6.7		
POMEGRANATE, raw (USDA) pulp only	4 oz.	.3		
POMPANO, raw (USDA) meat only	4 oz.	10.8		
PONDEROSA STEAKHOUSE :				
Beef, chopped, patty only:				
Regular	3½ oz.	10.8		
Double Deluxe	5.9 oz.	18.8		
Junior (Square Shooters)	1.6 oz.	5.1		
Steakhouse Deluxe	2.96 oz.	9.4		
Beverages:				
Coca-Cola	8 fl. oz.	0.0		
Dr Pepper	8 fl. oz.	0.0		
Milk, chocolate	8 fl. oz.	8.5		
Orange drink	8 fl. oz.	Tr.		
Root beer	8 fl. oz.	0.0		
Sprite	8 fl. oz.	0.0		
Tab	8 fl. oz.	0.0		
Bun:				
Regular	2.4-oz. bun	3.0		
Hot dog	1 bun	1.8		
Steakhouse deluxe	2.4-oz. bun	3.0		
Cocktail sauce	1½ oz.	.3		
Filet mignon	3.8 oz. (edible portion)	8.3		
Filet of sole, fish only (See also Bun)	3-oz. piece	4.9		
Fish, baked	4.9-oz. serving	13.5		
Gelatin dessert	½ cup	Tr.		
Gravy, au jus	1 oz.	.2		
Hot dog, child's, meat only (See also Bun)	1.6-oz. hot dog	13.0		
Margarine:				
Pat	1 tsp.	4.1		
On potato, as served	½ oz.	11.3		
Mustard sauce, sweet & sour	1 oz.	1.1		
New York strip steak	6.1 oz. (edible portion)	19.2		
Onion, chopped	1 T.	Tr.		
Pickle, dill	3 slices (.7 oz.)	Tr.		
Potato:				
Baked	7.2-oz. potato	.2		
French fries	3-oz. serving	11.1		
Pudding, chocolate	4½ oz.	10.6		
Ribeye	3.2 oz. (edible portion)	10.9		
Ribeye & shrimp:				
Ribeye	3.2 oz.	10.9		
Shrimp	2.2 oz.	6.7		
Roll, kaiser	2.2-oz. roll	3.4		
Salad dressing:				
Blue cheese	1 oz.	12.9		
Italian, creamy	1 oz.	12.9		
Low calorie	1 oz.	Tr.		
Oil & vinegar	1 oz.	13.8		
Thousand island	1 oz.	10.6		

FOOD DESCRIPTION	MEASURE OR QUANTITY	FATS IN GRAMS		
		Total	Saturated	Unsaturated
Shrimp dinner, shrimp only	7 pieces (3½ oz.)	10.6		
Steak sauce	1 oz.	.5		
Tartar sauce	1.5 oz.	3.0		
T-Bone	4.3 oz. (edible portion)	8.8		
Tomato:				
Slices	2 slices (.9 oz.)	Tr.		
Whole, small	3.5 oz.	.2		
Topping, whipped	¼ oz.	1.6		
Worcestershire sauce	1 tsp.	Tr.		
POPCORN:				
Unpopped (USDA)	1 oz.	1.3	Tr.	1.0
Popped, fresh:				
(Jolly Time) no added butter or salt:				
Regular	1 cup	.2		
Microwave, natural or butter flavor	1 cup	3.5		
(Orville Redenbacher's):				
Caramel crunch	1 oz.	7.0		
Hot-air corn	1 cup	.3		
Microwave:				
Regular, butter flavor, salted	1 cup	1.5		
Natural, without salt	1 cup	2.0		
Original, plain	1 cup	.3		
(Pillsbury) microwave:				
Regular	1 cup	4.5		
Butter flavor	1 cup	4.0		
Packaged:				
(Cape Cod):				
Regular or cheese	1 oz.	10.0		
Light	1 oz.	6.0		
(Eagle) plain	1 oz.	12.0		
(Weight Watchers):				
Lightly salted	.66-oz. pkg.	4.0		
White cheddar cheese	.66-oz. pkg.	6.0		
POPCORN POPPING OIL				
(Orville Redenbacher's) buttery flavor)	1 T. (.5 oz.)	14.0		
POPOVER:				
Home recipe (USDA)	1.4-oz. popover (2¾" dia. at top, ¼ cup batter)	3.7	1.0	2.0
*Mix (Flako)	2.3-oz. popover (⅙ pkg.)	4.8		
POP-UP (See **TOASTER CAKE**)				
PORGY, raw (USDA) meat only	4 oz.	3.9		
PORK, medium-fat:				
Fresh (USDA):				
All lean cuts:				
Lean only:				
Raw, diced	1 cup (8.2 oz.)	26.4	10.0	17.0
Raw, strips	1 cup (8.2 oz.)	26.3	10.0	17.0
Roasted, chopped	1 cup (5 oz.)	20.0	7.0	13.0
Boston butt:				
Raw	1 lb. (weighed with bone & skin)	104.1	37.0	67.0
Roasted, lean & fat	4 oz.	32.3	11.0	21.0
Roasted, lean only	4 oz.	16.2	6.0	10.0
Chop:				
Broiled, lean & fat	4-oz. chop (weighed with bone)	23.9	8.0	16.0
Broiled, lean & fat	3-oz. chop (weighed without bone)	26.9	9.0	18.0
Broiled, lean only	3-oz. chop (weighed without bone)	13.1	5.0	8.0
Fat, separable, cooked	1 oz.	23.6	9.0	15.0
Ham (See also **HAM**):				
Raw	1 lb. (weighed with bone & skin)	102.6	37.0	66.0
Roasted, lean & fat	4 oz.	34.7	12.0	22.0
Roasted, lean only	4 oz.	11.3	5.0	7.0

FOOD DESCRIPTION	MEASURE OR QUANTITY	FATS IN GRAMS		
		Total	Saturated	Unsaturated
Loin:				
Raw	1 lb. (weighed with bone)	89.0	32.0	57.0
Broiled, lean & fat	4 oz.	35.9	12.0	24.0
Broiled, lean only	4 oz.	17.5	7.0	11.0
Roasted, lean & fat	4 oz.	32.3	11.0	21.0
Roasted, lean only	4 oz.	16.1	6.0	10.0
Picnic:				
Raw	1 lb. (weighed with bone & skin)	92.2	33.0	59.0
Simmered, lean & fat	4 oz.	34.6	12.0	22.0
Simmered, lean only	4 oz.	11.1	5.0	7.0
Spareribs:				
Raw, with bone	1 lb. (weighed with bone)	89.7	32.0	58.0
Raw, without bone	1 lb. (weighed without bone)	150.6	54.0	97.0
Braised, lean & fat	4 oz.	44.1	16.0	28.0
Cured, light commercial cure:				
Bacon (see **BACON**)				
Boston butt (USDA):				
Raw	1 lb. (weighed with bone & skin)	101.7	37.0	65.0
Roasted, lean & fat	4 oz.	29.1	10.0	19.0
Roasted, lean only	4 oz.	15.6	7.0	9.0
Ham (See also **HAM**) (USDA):				
Raw	1 lb. (weighed with bone & skin)	89.7	32.0	58.0
Raw, lean only, ground	1 cup (6 oz.)	14.4	5.0	9.0
Roasted, lean & fat	4 oz.	25.1	9.0	16.0
Roasted, lean only:	4 oz.	10.0	3.0	7.0
Chopped	1 cup (4.9 oz.)	12.1	4.0	8.0
Diced	1 cup (5.2 oz.)	12.9	4.0	9.0
Ground	1 cup (3.8 oz.)	9.6	3.0	6.0
Picnic (USDA):				
Raw	1 lb. (weighed with bone & skin)	87.8	32.0	56.0
Roasted, lean & fat	4 oz.	28.6	10.0	18.0
Roasted, lean only	4 oz.	11.2	5.0	7.0
PORK, CANNED, chopped luncheon meat (USDA)	1 cup (4.8 oz.)	33.9	12.0	22.0
PORK DINNER OR ENTREE:				
Canned (Hunt's) *Minute Gourmet* microwave entree maker, cajun:				
Without pork	3.9 oz.	1.0		
*With pork	6.6 oz.	23.0		
Frozen (Swanson) loin of	11¼-oz. dinner	11.0		
PORK RINDS, fried, *Baken-ets*	1 oz.	7.4	3.0	5.0
PORK SAUSAGE (See **SAUSAGE,** Pork)				
PORT WINE	Any quantity	0.0		
POSTUM, instant	1 cup (6 oz.)	Tr.		
POTATO:				
Raw (USDA):				
Whole	1 lb. (weighed unpared)	.4		
Pared:				
Chopped or slices	1 cup (5.2 oz.)	.1		
Diced	1 cup (5.5 oz.)	.2		
Cooked (USDA):				
Au gratin or scalloped:				
Without cheese	½ cup (4.3 oz.)	4.8	2.0	2.0
With cheese	½ cup (4.3 oz.)	9.6	5.0	5.0
Baked, peeled after baking, salted or unsalted	2½" dia. potato (3.5 oz., 3 raw per lb.)	.1		
Boiled, peeled before boiling, salted or unsalted:				
Whole	4.3-oz. potato (3 raw per lb.)	.1		
Diced or sliced	½ cup	Tr.		
Mashed or riced	½ cup	.1		

FOOD DESCRIPTION	MEASURE OR QUANTITY	FATS IN GRAMS		
		Total	Saturated	Unsaturated
French-fried in deep fat, salted or unsalted	10 pieces (2″ × ½″ × ½″, 2 oz.)	7.5	2.0	6.0
Hash-browned	½ cup (3.4 oz.)	11.4	3.0	8.0
Mashed:				
Milk added	½ cup (3.5 oz.)	.7		
Milk & butter added	½ cup (3.5 oz.)	4.2	2.0	2.0
Pan-fried from raw	½ cup (3 oz.)	12.1	3.0	10.0
Scalloped (See Au gratin)				
Canned, solids & liq.:				
(Allen) *Butterfield*	½ cup (4 oz.)	Tr.		
(Larsen) *Freshlike*	½ cup (4.5 oz.)	0.0		
Dehydrated, mashed (USDA):				
Flakes:				
Dry	½ cup (.8 oz.)	.1		
*Prepared with water, milk & butter	½ cup (3.8 oz.)	3.4	2.0	1.0
Granules, without milk:				
Dry	½ cup	.6		
*Prepared with water, milk & butter	½ cup (3.7 oz.)	3.8	2.0	2.0
Frozen:				
(Birds Eye):				
Cottage fries	¼ of 14-oz. pkg.	4.2		
Crinkle cuts, regular	3 oz.	3.8		
French fries, *Deep Gold*	3 oz.	6.0		
Hash browns, shredded	3 oz.	.3		
Shoestring	3 oz.	5.2		
Whole, peeled	1/10 of 32-oz. pkg.	Tr.		
(Empire Kosher) french fries	3 oz.	4.0		
(Green Giant) One serving:				
Au gratin	5½-oz. serving	10.0	4.0	2.0
& broccoli in cheese sauce	5½-oz. serving	5.0	Tr.	2.0
(Larsen) diced	4 oz.	0.0		
(Ore-Ida):				
Cheddar Browns	3 oz.	2.0	1.0	Tr.
Cottage fries	3 oz.	5.0	Tr.	3.0
Country Style Dinner Fries or *Home Style Potato Wedges*	3 oz.	3.0	Tr.	<3.0
Crinkle cuts:				
Deep fries	3 oz.	6.0	1.0	<5.0
Microwave	3½ oz.	8.0	1.0	6.0
Crispers	3 oz.	15.0	3.0	12.0
Crispy Crowns	3 oz.	10.0	2.0	8.0
Golden Crinkles	3 oz.	5.0	Tr.	<4.0
Hash browns:				
Microwave	2 oz.	7.0	1.0	<6.0
Shredded	3 oz.	40.0		
Toaster	1¾ oz.	6.0	4.0	<4.0
Potatoes O'Brien	3 oz.	Tr.	Tr.	Tr.
Shoestrings	3 oz.	6.0	Tr.	<5.0
Tater Tots:				
Plain:				
Regular	3 oz.	7.0	1.0	<6.0
Microwave	4 oz.	9.0	2.0	7.0
Bacon flavored	3 oz.	7.0	1.0	<6.0
Whole, small, peeled	3 oz.	Tr.	Tr.	Tr.
POTATO CHIP:				
(Cape Cod) any type	1 oz.	8.0		
(Cottage Fries) no salt added	1 oz.	11.0		
(Eagle):				
BBQ:				
Crunchy or Louisiana	1 oz.	8.0		
Thins	1 oz.	10.0		
Ridged, sour cream & onion, or thins	1 oz.	10.0		

FOOD DESCRIPTION	MEASURE OR QUANTITY	FATS IN GRAMS		
		Total	Saturated	Unsaturated
(Lay's):				
Regular, sour cream & onion, or unsalted	1 oz.	10.0		
BBQ, Italian cheese, jalapeño & cheddar, or salt & vinegar	1 oz.	9.0		
(New York Deli)	1 oz.	11.0		
(Pringle's):				
Regular or sour cream & onion	1 oz.	13.1		
Cheese-Umms	1 oz.	13.0		
Light style	1 oz.	8.2		
(Ruffles) regular or cajun spice	1 oz.	10.0		
POTATO MIX:				
*Au gratin (Betty Crocker)	⅙ of pkg.	5.0		
*Casserole (French's) with cheddar cheese & bacon	½ cup	5.0		
Cheddar bacon:				
*(Betty Crocker)	⅙ of pkg.	5.0		
(Lipton) & sauce	½ cup	1.3		
*Hash browns (Betty Crocker) with onions	½ cup	6.0		
*Julienne (Betty Crocker)	½ cup	5.0		
Mashed:				
*(Betty Crocker) *Buds*	½ cup	6.0		
(Borden) *Country Store*	⅓ cup flakes	0.0		
*(French's) Idaho, regular	½ cup	6.0		
*Scalloped (Betty Crocker) plain or cheesy	½ cup	5.0		
*Sour cream & chive (French's)	½ cup	7.0		
*Stroganoff (French's)	½ cup	4.0		
*POTATO PANCAKE MIX (French's)	3″ pancake	.7		
POTATO SALAD, home recipe (USDA):				
Cooked salad dressing & seasonings	4 oz.	3.2	1.0	2.0
With mayonnaise & French dressing, hard-cooked eggs & seasonings	½ cup (4.4 oz.)	11.5	2.0	9.0
POTATO STICK (Durkee) *O & C*	1½ oz.	15.0		
POTATO, STUFFED, BAKED:				
*Mix (Betty Crocker):				
Bacon & cheese, mild cheddar with onion or sour cream & chive	⅙ of pkg.	11.0		
Herbed butter	⅙ of pkg.	13.0		
Frozen:				
(Ore-Ida):				
Butter flavor or sour cream & chive	5-oz. serving	9.0	2.0	6.0
Cheddar cheese	5-oz. serving	11.0	3.0	7.0
(Weight Watchers):				
Broccoli & cheese	10½-oz. pkg.	7.0	4.0	3.0
Chicken divan	11-oz. pkg.	4.0	2.0	<3.0
POT ROAST DINNER OR ENTREE, frozen:				
(Armour) *Dinner Classics,* yankee	10-oz. meal	12.0		
(Healthy Choice) yankee	11-oz. meal	4.0	2.0	Tr.
(Stouffer's) *Right Course*	9¼-oz. meal	7.0		
POUND CAKE (See **CAKE,** Pound)				
PRESERVE, sweetened (See also individual listings by flavor) (USDA)	1 T. (.7 oz.)	Tr.		

FOOD DESCRIPTION	MEASURE OR QUANTITY	Total	Saturated	Unsaturated
PRETZEL:				
(Eagle Snacks)	1 oz.	2.0		
Mister Salty (Nabisco):				
Regular:				
Dutch or rods	1 piece	.5		
Nuggets	1 piece	Tr.		
Sticks, *Veri-Thin*	1 piece	Tr.		
Twists	1 piece	.4		
Juniors	1 piece	Tr.		
(Snyder's) hard	1 oz.	7.1		
PRICKLY PEAR, fresh (USDA)				
flesh only	4 oz.	.1		
PRODUCT 19, cereal				
(Kellogg's)	1 cup (1 oz.)	0.0		
PROSCIUTTO (Hormel)				
boneless	1 oz.	7.0		
PRUNE:				
Dried, "softenized," uncooked (USDA):				
Small	1 prune (5 grams)	Tr.		
Large	1 prune (9 grams)	Tr.		
Pitted:				
Chopped	1 cup (5.3 oz.)	.9		
Ground	1 cup (9.7 oz.)	1.6		
Dried, moist-pak (Del Monte)	1 cup (8 oz.)	.9		
Dried, ready-to-eat (Del Monte)	1 cup (6.6 oz.)	4.7		
Dried, softenized, cooked, unsweetened (USDA)	1 cup (17–18 med. with 1/3 cup liq., 9.5 oz.)	.7		
Dried, softenized, cooked with sugar (USDA)	1 cup (16–18 prunes & 1/3 cup liq., 11.1 oz.)	.6		
Dehydrated (USDA):				
Nugget-type & pieces	8 oz.	1.1		
Nugget-type & pieces, cooked with sugar, solids & liq.	1 cup (8.9 oz.)	.5		
Canned:				
Cooked (Sunsweet)	1 cup	.4		
Stewed, pitted (Del Monte)	1 cup (9.2 oz.)	1.3		
PRUNE JUICE (Sunsweet)	6 fl. oz.	Tr.		
PRUNE WHIP, home recipe (USDA)	1 cup (4.8 oz.)	.3		
PUDDING OR PIE FILLING:				
Home recipe (USDA):				
Chocolate	1/2 cup (4.6 oz.)	6.9		
Rice, with raisins	1/2 cup (4.7 oz.)	4.1	2.6	1.5
Tapioca:				
Apple	1/2 cup (4.4 oz.)	.1		
Cream	1/2 cup (2.9 oz.)	4.2		
Vanilla, blancmange	1/2 cup (4.5 oz.)	5.0		
Canned, regular pack:				
Banana:				
(Hunt's) *Snack Pack*	4 1/4 oz.	9.0		
(Thank You Brand)	1/2 cup (4.6 oz.)	3.9		
Butterscotch:				
(Hunt's) *Snack Pack*	4 1/4 oz.	8.0		
(Thank You Brand)	1/2 cup (4.6 oz.)	3.9		
Chocolate:				
(Hunt's) *Snack Pack:*				
Regular, German or marshmallows	4 1/4 oz.	7.0		
Fudge	4 1/4 oz.	9.0		
(Thank You Brand) fudge	1/2 cup (4.6 oz.)	3.9		
Lemon (Hunt's) *Snack Pack*	4 1/4 oz.	3.0		
Rice:				
(Comstock)	3 3/4 oz.	3.0		
(Hunt's) *Snack Pack*	4 1/4 oz.	10.0		

FOOD DESCRIPTION	MEASURE OR QUANTITY	FATS IN GRAMS		
		Total	Saturated	Unsaturated
Tapioca:				
(Hunt's) *Snack Pack*	4¼ oz.	5.0		
(Swiss Miss)	4 oz.	4.0		
Vanilla:				
(Hunt's) *Snack Pack*	4¼ oz.	7.0		
(Swiss Miss)	4 oz.	6.0		
Canned, dietetic (Estee) any flavor	½ cup	Tr.		
*Mix, regular:				
Banana, cream:				
(Jell-O) regular or instant	½ cup	4.2		
(Royal) regular	½ cup	4.0		
Butter pecan (Jell-O) instant	½ cup	4.9		
Butterscotch:				
(Jell-O) regular or instant	½ cup	4.3		
(Royal) regular	½ cup	4.0		
Chocolate:				
(Jell-O) any flavor, regular or instant	½ cup	4.4		
(Royal) plain, regular or instant	½ cup	4.0		
Coconut:				
(Jell-O) cream, regular	½ cup	6.6		
(Royal) toasted, instant	½ cup	4.0		
Custard:				
(Jell-O)	½ cup	5.0		
(Royal)	½ cup	5.0		
Flan (Knorr) with or without sauce	½ cup	4.0		
Lemon:				
(Jell-O):				
Regular	½ cup	1.9		
Instant	½ cup	4.3		
(Royal) instant	½ cup	5.0		
Lime (Royal) regular	½ cup	3.0		
Pistachio (Jell-O) instant	½ cup	4.9		
Rice (Jell-O)	½ cup	4.1		
Tapioca:				
(Jell-O)	½ cup	4.0		
(Royal) vanilla	½ cup	1.0		
Vanilla:				
(Jell-O) regular or instant	½ cup	4.0		
(Royal) regular	½ cup	4.0		
*Mix, dietetic:				
Butterscotch:				
(D-Zerta)	½ cup	Tr.		
(Weight Watchers)	½ cup	0.0		
Chocolate:				
(Estee) instant	½ cup	Tr.		
(Weight Watchers)	½ cup	1.0		
Vanilla:				
(Estee)	½ cup	Tr.		
(Weight Watchers)	½ cup	0.0		
PUDDING STIX (Good Humor)	1¾-fl.-oz. pop	2.0		
PUDDING SUNDAE (Swiss Miss):				
Chocolate	4 oz.	7.0		
Mint or peanut butter	4 oz.	11.0		
PUFF (See **CRACKER** or individual kinds of hors d'oeuvres, such as **CHICKEN PUFF**)				
PUFFED OAT CEREAL				
(USDA):				
Added nutrients	1 oz.	1.6		
Sugar-coated, added nutrients	1 oz.	1.0		
PUFFED RICE CEREAL:				
(Malt-O-Meal)	½ cup	.2		
(Quaker)	1 cup (½ oz.)	.1		

FOOD DESCRIPTION	MEASURE OR QUANTITY	FATS IN GRAMS		
		Total	Saturated	Unsaturated
PUMPKIN:				
Fresh (USDA) flesh only	4 oz.	.1		
Canned:				
(Del Monte)	½ cup	0.0		
(Libby's)	½ cup (4.1 oz.)	.5		
PUMPKIN SEED, dry (USDA) hulled	3 oz.	53.0	9.0	44.0
PURE & LIGHT, canned (Dole) fruit juice, any flavor	6 fl. oz.	0.0		
QUAIL, raw (USDA):				
Meat & skin only	4 oz.	7.9		
Giblets	2 oz.	3.5		
QUIK (Nestlé) any flavor	1 tsp.	Tr.		
RABBIT (USDA):				
Domesticated:				
Ready-to-cook	1 lb. (weighed with bones)	29.0	11.0	18.0
Stewed, flesh only	4 oz.	11.5		
Stewed, flesh only, chopped or diced	1 cup (4.9 oz.)	14.1		
Wild, ready-to-cook	1 lb. (weighed with bones)	18.1		
RACCOON, roasted, meat only (USDA)	4 oz.	16.4		
RADISH (USDA):				
Common, raw:				
Untrimmed, without tops	⅓ lb. (weighed untrimmed)	.2		
Trimmed, whole	4 small radishes (1.4 oz.)	Tr.		
Oriental, raw, trimmed & pared	3 oz.	.1		
RAISIN:				
Dried:				
Whole (USDA)	4 oz.	.2		
Whole (USDA)	.5-oz. pkg.	Tr.		
Chopped (USDA)	½ cup (2.9 oz.)	.2		
Ground (USDA)	½ cup (4.7 oz.)	.3		
Seedless:				
(Del Monte) golden	3 oz.	0.0		
(Sun-Maid) California Thompson	3 oz.	0.0		
Cooked, added sugar (USDA) solids & liq.	½ cup (4.3 oz.)	.1		
RASPBERRY:				
Black (USDA):				
Fresh:				
Whole	½ lb. (weighed with caps & stems)	3.1		
Without caps & stems	½ cup (2.4 oz.)	.9		
Canned, water pack, un-sweetened, solids & liq.	4 oz.	1.2		
Red:				
Fresh (USDA):				
Whole	½ lb. (weighed with caps & stems)	1.1		
Without caps & stems	½ cup (2.5 oz.)	.4		
Canned, water pack, un-sweetened or low-calorie, solids & liq.:				
(USDA)	4 oz.	.1		
(Blue Boy)	4 oz.	1.0		
Frozen, sweetened (Birds Eye) quick thaw	½ cup (5 oz.)	.2		
*RASPBERRY DRINK,** mix (Funny Face)	8 fl. oz.	0.0		
RASPBERRY PRESERVE OR JAM:				
Sweetened (Bama)	1 T. (.7 oz.)	Tr.		
Low-calorie or dietetic (Estee)	1 T.	0.0		
RATATOUILLE, frozen (Stouffer's)	5 oz.	3.0		

FOOD DESCRIPTION	MEASURE OR QUANTITY	FATS IN GRAMS		
		Total	Saturated	Unsaturated
RAVIOLI:				
Canned, regular pack (Franco-American) beef:				
In meat sauce	7½-oz. can	5.0		
In meat sauce, *RavioliOs*	7½-oz. can	7.0		
Canned, dietetic:				
(Dia-Mel) beef	8 oz.	10.0		
(Estee) beef	7½-oz. can	8.0		
Frozen:				
(Celentano) cheese:				
Regular size	½ of 13-oz. pkg.	11.0		
Mini	½ of 8-oz. pkg.	5.0		
(Kid Cuisine) cheese, mini	8¾-oz. meal	2.0		
(Weight Watchers) cheese, baked	8⅙-oz. pkg.	12.0	5.0	7.0
RED & GRAY SNAPPER, raw (USDA) meat only	4 oz.	1.0		
RED LOBSTER (All "lunch portions" weigh 5 oz. before cooking):				
Calamari, breaded & fried	1 lunch portion	21.0		
Catfish	1 lunch portion	10.0		
Chicken breast	4-oz. serving	3.0		
Clam, cherrystone	1 order	2.0		
Cod, Atlantic	1 lunch portion	1.0		
Crab legs, king or snow	16-oz. serving	2.0		
Flounder	1 lunch portion	1.0		
Grouper	1 lunch portion	1.0		
Haddock	1 lunch portion	1.0		
Halibut	1 lunch portion	1.0		
Hamburger patty, no bun	5.3-oz. serving	23.0		
Lobster tail, rock	1 tail	3.0		
Mackerel	1 lunch portion	12.0		
Mussels	3-oz. serving	2.0		
Oysters	6 raw oysters	4.0		
Perch, ocean	1 lunch portion	4.0		
Pollock	1 lunch portion	1.0		
Rockfish, red	1 lunch portion	1.0		
Salmon:				
Norwegian	1 lunch portion	12.0		
Sockeye	1 lunch portion	4.0		
Scallop, calico or deep sea	1 lunch portion	2.0		
Shark, blacktip or mako	1 lunch portion	1.0		
Shrimp	8–12 pieces	2.0		
Snapper, red	1 lunch portion	1.0		
Sole, lemon	1 lunch portion	1.0		
Steak:				
Porterhouse	18-oz. steak	131.0		
Sirloin	7-oz. steak	48.0		
Strip	7-oz. steak	64.0		
Swordfish	1 lunch portion	4.0		
Tuna, yellowfin	1 lunch portion	6.0		
REINDEER, raw, lean only (USDA)	4 oz.	4.3		
RELISH:				
Dill (Vlasic)	1 oz.	0.0		
Hamburger (Vlasic)	1 oz.	0.0		
Hot dog (Vlasic)	1 oz.	0.0		
Sour (USDA)	1 T. (.5 oz.)	.1		
Sweet (Vlasic)	1 oz.	0.0		
RENNETT MIX (Junket):				
*Powder, chocolate, raspberry or strawberry:				
Made with skim milk	½ cup	0.0		
Made with whole milk	½ cup	4.0		
*Tablet:				
Made with skim milk	½ cup	0.0		
Made with whole milk	½ cup	4.0		
RHINE WINE	Any quantity	0.0		

FOOD DESCRIPTION	MEASURE OR QUANTITY	FATS IN GRAMS		
		Total	Saturated	Unsaturated
RHUBARB:				
Fresh (USDA):				
Trimmed	4 oz.	.1		
Diced	½ cup (2.2 oz.)	Tr.		
Cooked, sweetened (USDA)				
solids & liq.	½ cup (4.2 oz.)	.1		
Frozen, sweetened:				
(USDA) cooked, added				
sugar, solids & liq.	½ cup (4.4 oz.)	.2		
(Birds Eye)	½ cup (4 oz.)	.1		
RICE:				
Brown:				
Raw (USDA)	½ cup (3.7 oz.)	2.0		
Raw (USDA)	1 oz.	.5		
Cooked, with added salt:				
(Carolina)	4 oz.	.7		
(Uncle Ben's) parboiled:				
With no added butter	⅔ cup (4.2 oz.)	1.1		
With added butter	⅔ cup (4.3 oz.)	3.2		
White:				
Instant or precooked:				
Dry, long-grain (USDA)	½ cup (1.9 oz.)	.1		
Cooked, with or without salt:				
(USDA) long-grain	⅔ cup (3.3 oz.)	Tr.		
(Minute Rice) no added butter	⅔ cup (4 oz.)	Tr.		
(Uncle Ben's) long-grain:				
No added butter	⅔ cup (4 oz.)	Tr.		
Added butter	⅔ cup (4.1 oz.)	2.5		
Parboiled:				
Dry, long-grain (USDA)	1 oz.	Tr.		
Cooked, with or without added salt:				
(USDA) long-grain, added salt	⅔ cup (4.1 oz.)	.1		
(Aunt Carolina)	⅔ cup (4.1 oz.)	.1		
Wild (See **WILD RICE**)				
RICE BRAN (USDA)	1 oz.	Tr.		
RICE CAKE:				
(Hain):				
Regular	1 cake	Tr.		
Mini:				
Plain, apple cinnamon, teriyaki	1 cake	Tr.		
Barbecue	1 cake	3.0		
Cheese, nacho cheese or ranch	1 cake	2.0		
Heart Lovers (TKI Foods) plain or sesame	1 cake (.3 oz.)	0.0		
(Pritikin) any flavor	1 cake	0.0		
RICE, FRIED (See also **RICE MIX**):				
*Canned (La Choy)	⅓ of 11-oz. can	2.0		
Frozen:				
(Birds Eye)	⅓ of 11-oz. pkg.	.3		
(La Choy) with meat	8-oz. entree	4.0		
Seasoning mix (Kikkoman)	1-oz. pkg.	.2		
RICE KRISPIES, cereal				
(Kellogg's) any flavor	1 oz.	0.0		
RICE MIX:				
Beef:				
(Lipton) & sauce	½ cup	.5		
*(Minute Rice) rib roast	½ cup	4.1		
Chicken:				
(Lipton) & sauce	¼ of pkg.	1.1		
*(Minute Rice)	½ cup	4.3		
*Fried (Minute Rice)	½ cup	4.3		

FOOD DESCRIPTION	MEASURE OR QUANTITY	FATS IN GRAMS		
		Total	Saturated	Unsaturated
*Long-grain & wild (Minute Rice)	½ cup	4.1		
*Milanese (Knorr) risotto	½ cup	3.0		
Spanish (See also **RICE, SPANISH**):				
*(Lipton) & sauce	½ cup	3.0		
*(Minute Rice)	½ cup	4.1		
RICE, POLISH (USDA)	1 oz.	3.6		
***RICE SEASONING** (French's)				
Spice Your Rice:				
Beef flavor & onion, cheese'n chives, chicken flavor & herb or chicken flavor & parmesan	½ cup	4.0		
Buttery herb	½ cup	5.0		
RICE, SPANISH:				
Home recipe (USDA)	4 oz.	1.9		
Canned (Old El Paso)	½ cup	1.0	0.0	0.0
Frozen (Birds Eye)	⅓ of 11-oz. pkg.	.5		
RICE & VEGETABLE:				
Frozen:				
(Birds Eye):				
For one:				
& broccoli, au gratin	5¾-oz. pkg.	10.0		
& green beans & almonds	5½-oz. pkg.	10.0		
Pilaf	5½-oz. pkg.	9.4		
Internationals:				
Country or French style	⅓ of 10-oz. pkg.	Tr.		
Spanish style	⅓ of 10-oz. pkg.	1.0		
(Green Giant):				
One serving:				
& broccoli in cheese sauce	4½-oz. pkg.	6.0	2.0	1.0
With peas & mushrooms	5½-oz. pkg.	2.0	Tr.	0.0
Rice Originals:				
& broccoli, in cheese sauce	½ cup (4 oz.)	4.0	1.0	Tr.
Italian blend & spinach in cheese sauce	½ cup (4 oz.)	4.0	3.0	Tr.
Pilaf	½ cup (4 oz.)	1.0	Tr.	0.0
Mix:				
*(Knorr) any flavor	½ cup	3.0		
(Lipton) & sauce:				
Asparagus with hollandaise sauce	½ cup	.9		
& broccoli with cheddar cheese	½ cup	1.7		
RIGATONI, frozen (Healthy Choice) & meat sauce	9½-oz. serving	4.0	2.0	Tr.
ROCKFISH (USDA) oven steamed, with onion	4 oz.	2.8		
ROE (USDA):				
Baked or broiled with butter or margarine & lemon juice or vinegar, cod & shad	4 oz.	3.2		
Canned, cod, haddock or herring, solids & liq.	4 oz.	3.2		
ROLL & BUN:				
Commercial-type, non-frozen:				
Apple (Dolly Madison)	2-oz. bun	4.0		
Brown & serve:				
Merita (Interstate Brands)	1-oz. roll	1.0		
(Pepperidge Farm)	1.3-oz. roll	1.0		
(Roman Meal) original	1-oz. roll	1.8		
Cinnamon (Dolly Madison)	1¾-oz. roll	6.0		

FOOD DESCRIPTION	MEASURE OR QUANTITY	Total	Saturated	Unsaturated
Cloverleaf (USDA) home recipe	1.2-oz. roll	3.0	.7	2.3
Crescent (Pepperidge Farm) butter	1-oz. roll	6.0		
Croissant (Pepperidge Farm):				
Butter	2-oz. roll	13.0		
Chocolate	2.4-oz. roll	16.0		
Raisin	2-oz. roll	10.0		
Danish (Dolly Madison) *Danish Twirls:*				
Apple	2-oz. roll	13.0		
Cherry	2-oz. roll	12.0		
Cinnamon raisin	2-oz. roll	14.0		
Dinner:				
Butternut	1-oz. roll	2.0		
Holsum	2-oz. roll	4.0		
(Roman Meal) original	1½-oz. roll	2.3	.1	
French:				
(Arnold) *Francisco*	1.1-oz. roll	1.0		
(Pepperidge Farm)	1.3-oz. roll	2.0		
Golden twist (Pepperidge Farm)	1-oz. roll	6.0		
Hamburger:				
(Arnold)	1.4-oz. roll	1.0		
(Roman Meal) original	1.6-oz. roll	2.5		
Hard (USDA) round or rectangular	1.8-oz. roll	1.6	.5	1.1
Honey (Dolly Madison)	3½-oz. bun	24.0		
Lemon (Dolly Madison)	2-oz. bun	5.0		
Parker House (Pepperidge Farm)	.6-oz. roll	1.0		
Raspberry (Dolly Madison)	2-oz. bun	6.0		
Sourdough French (Pepperidge Farm)	1.3-oz. roll	2.0		
Steak, *Butternut*	1.5-oz. roll	2.0		
ROLL OR BUN DOUGH:				
Frozen:				
(USDA):				
Unbaked	1 oz.	1.4	Tr.	1.0
Baked	1 oz.	1.5	Tr.	1.0
*(Rich's) home-style	1 roll	1.0		
*Refrigerated:				
(Pillsbury):				
Butterflake	1 piece	5.0	2.0	Tr.
Caramel danish with nuts	1 piece	8.0	3.0	Tr.
Cinnamon:				
Plain	1 piece	9.0	3.0	Tr.
With icing:				
Regular	1 piece	4.5	1.0	0.0
& raisin danish	1 piece	7.0	2.0	Tr.
Crescent	1 piece	5.5	2.0	0.0
(Roman Meal):				
Regular	1.2-oz. piece	1.9		
Honey nut oat bran or white	1½-oz. piece	4.7		
ROLL MIX:				
(USDA):				
Dry mix	1 oz.	1.7	Tr.	1.0
*Prepared with water	1 oz.	1.3	Tr.	1.0
(Pillsbury) hot	1 oz.	2.0		
ROSÉ WINE	Any quantity	0.0		
ROY ROGERS:				
Bar Burger, R.R.	1 burger	31.0		
Biscuit	1 biscuit	12.1		
Breakfast crescent sandwich:				
Regular	4.5-oz. sandwich	27.0		
With bacon	4.7-oz. sandwich	29.7		
With ham	5.8-oz. sandwich	29.0		
With sausage	5.7-oz. sandwich	42.0		

FOOD DESCRIPTION	MEASURE OR QUANTITY	FATS IN GRAMS		
		Total	Saturated	Unsaturated
Cheeseburger:				
Regular	1 burger	29.0		
With bacon	1 burger	33.0		
Chicken:				
Breast	1 piece	23.7		
Leg	1 piece	8.0		
Thigh	1 piece	19.5		
Wing	1 piece	12.8		
Chicken nuggets	1 piece	6.0		
Coleslaw	3½-oz. serving	6.0		
Drinks:				
Coffee, black	6 fl. oz.	Tr.		
Coca-Cola, regular or diet	Any quantity	0.0		
Hot chocolate	6 fl. oz.	2.0		
Milk	8 fl. oz.	8.2		
Orange juice	7 fl. oz.	.2		
Shake:				
Chocolate or strawberry	1 shake	10.2		
Vanilla	1 shake	10.7		
Tea, iced, plain	8 fl. oz.	0.0		
Egg & biscuit platter:				
Regular	1 serving	34.0		
With bacon	1 serving	39.0		
With ham	1 serving	36.0		
With sausage	1 serving	49.0		
Hamburger	1 burger	25.0		
Pancake platter, with syrup & butter:				
Plain	1 serving	13.0		
With bacon	1 serving	17.0		
With ham	1 serving	15.0		
With sausage	1 serving	28.0		
Potato, french fries:				
Regular order	3 oz.	12.0		
Large order	4 oz.	16.0		
Potato salad	3½-oz. order	6.1		
Roast beef sandwich:				
Plain:				
Regular	1 sandwich	11.0		
Large	1 sandwich	11.9		
With cheese:				
Regular	1 sandwich	15.0		
Large	1 sandwich	17.0		
Salad dressing:				
Regular:				
Bacon & tomato	1 T.	6.0		
Bleu cheese	1 T.	8.0		
Ranch	1 T.	7.0		
Thousand island	1 T.	8.0		
Low-calorie, Italian	1 T.	3.0		
Strawberry shortcake	7.2-oz. serving	19.2		
Sundae:				
Caramel	1 sundae	8.5		
Hot fudge	1 sundae	12.5		
Strawberry	1 sundae	7.1		
RUSK (USDA)	1 piece (.5 oz.)	1.2	Tr.	1.0
RUTABAGA:				
Raw (USDA) diced	½ cup (2.5 oz.)	Tr.		
Boiled, without salt (USDA) diced, drained	½ cup (3 oz.)	Tr.		
Canned (Sunshine) solids & liq.	½ cup (4.2 oz.)	.1		
Frozen (Southland)	4 oz.	0.0		
RYE, whole grain (USDA)	1 oz.	.5		
RYE WHISKEY (See **DISTILLED LIQUOR**)				
RYKRISP (See **CRACKER**)				
SABLEFISH, raw (USDA) meat only	4 oz.	16.9		

FOOD DESCRIPTION	MEASURE OR QUANTITY	FATS IN GRAMS		
		Total	Saturated	Unsaturated
SAFFLOWER SEED (USDA):				
Kernels, dry, hulled	1 oz.	16.9	1.0	15.0
Meal, partially defatted	1 oz.	2.3	Tr.	2.0
SALAD DRESSING:				
Regular:				
Bacon & tomato (Henri's)	1 T. (.5 oz.)	6.0		
Bleu or blue cheese				
(Henri's)	1 T. (.5 oz.)	5.0		
Buttermilk (Hain)	1 T.	7.0		
Caesar:				
(Hain) creamy	1 T.	6.0		
(Wish-Bone)	1 T.	8.1		
Cucumber dill (Hain)	1 T.	8.0		
Dijon vinaigrette:				
(Hain)	1 T.	5.0		
(Wish-Bone)	1 T.	6.1		
French:				
(Henri's) any type	1 T.	6.0		
(Wish-Bone)	1 T.	5.5		
Garlic (Wish-Bone) creamy	1 T.	8.0		
Honey & sesame (Hain)	1 T.	5.0		
Italian:				
(Hain):				
Canola oil	1 T.	5.0		
Creamy or traditional	1 T.	8.0		
(Henri's):				
Authentic	1 T.	8.0		
Creamy garlic	1 T.	5.0		
(Wish-Bone):				
Creamy	1 T.	5.4		
Herbal or robusto	1 T.	7.3		
Mayonnaise-type, *Blue Plate* (Luzianne)	1 T.	6.0		
Poppyseed rancher's (Hain)	1 T.	7.0		
Ranch (Henri's) *Chef's Recipe* or parmesan	1 T.	7.0		
Red wine vinaigrette (Wish-Bone)	1 T.	3.6		
Russian:				
(Henri's)	1 T.	5.0		
(Wish-Bone)	1 T.	2.5		
Sour cream & bacon (Wish-Bone)	1 T.	7.0		
Tas-Tee (Henri's)	1 T.	5.0		
Thousand island:				
(Hain)	1 T.	5.0		
(Wish-Bone)	1 T.	5.6		
Dietetic:				
Bleu cheese:				
(Estee)	1 T.	Tr.	Tr.	
(Henri's)	1 T.	2.0		
(Wish-Bone) chunky	1 T.	4.0		
Caesar (Hain)	1 T.	1.0		
Cucumber & onion				
(Henri's)	1 T.	2.0		
Dijon (Estee) creamy	1 T.	Tr.		
French:				
(Henri's)	1 T.	2.0		
(Pritikin)	1 T.	0.0		
Garlic (Estee) creamy	1 T.	0.0		
Herb (Hain)	1 T.	10.0		
Herb basket, *Herb Magic* (Luzianne Blue Plate)	1 T.	0.0		
Italian:				
(Estee) creamy	1 T.	0.0		
(Hain) creamy	1 T.	8.0		
(Henri's)	1 T.	2.0		
(Pritikin)	1 T.	0.0		
(Weight Watchers)	1 T. (.5 oz.)	5.0	1.0	3.0

FOOD DESCRIPTION	MEASURE OR QUANTITY	FATS IN GRAMS		
		Total	Saturated	Unsaturated
Olive oil vinaigrette (Wish-Bone) lite	1 T.	.9		
Ranch:				
(Pritikin)	1 T.	0.0		
(Weight Watchers)	3/4-oz. packet	0.0		
(Wish-Bone)	1 T.	3.5		
Red wine vinegar (Estee)	1 T.	0.0		
Russian:				
(Pritikin)	1 T.	0.0		
(Weight Watchers)	1 T.	5.0	1.0	3.0
(Wish-Bone)	1 T.	Tr.		
Thousand island:				
(Estee)	1 T.	0.0		
(Henri's)	1 T.	2.0		
(Weight Watchers)	1 T.	5.0	1.0	3.0
Vinaigrette:				
Herb Magic (Luzianne Blue Plate)	1 T.	0.0		
(Pritikin)	1 T.	0.0		
Whipped (Weight Watchers)	1 T.	4.0	1.0	2.0
*SALAD DRESSING MIX:				
Regular (Good Seasons):				
Bleu cheese, garlic, garlic & herbs, Italian, or lemon & herbs	1 T.	8.0		
Buttermilk or ranch	1 T.	6.0		
Classic dill	1 T.	7.7	2.2	6.2
Dietetic:				
Bleu cheese (Hain) no oil	1 T.	1.0		
Caesar (Hain)	1 T.	Tr.		
French (Hain)	1 T.	0.0		
Italian:				
(Good Seasons):				
Lite	1 T.	3.0		
No oil	1 T.	Tr.		
(Hain) no oil	1 T.	0.0		
Ranch (Hain) lite	1 T.	2.0		
1000 Island (Hain)	1 T.	0.0		
SALAMI:				
(USDA):				
Dry	1 oz.	10.8		
Cooked	1 oz.	7.3		
(Eckrich):				
For beer or cooked	1 oz.	6.0		
Cotto, meat	1-oz. slice	5.0		
Hard	1 oz.	12.0		
(Hormel):				
Beef	1 slice	25.0		
Genoa:				
Di Lusso	1 oz.	8.0		
San Remo Brand	1 oz.	10.0		
Hard:				
Packaged, sliced	1 slice	3.5		
Whole, regular	1 oz.	10.0		
(Oscar Mayer):				
For beer, regular	.8-oz. slice	4.0	1.7	2.9
Genoa or hard	.3-oz. slice	2.0	1.2	1.7
SALISBURY STEAK, frozen:				
(Armour):				
Classics Lite	11½-oz. meal	11.0		
Dinner Classics:				
Regular	11¼-oz. meal	17.0		
Parmigiana	11½-oz. meal	21.0		
(Banquet) dinner, regular	11-oz. meal	34.0		
(Healthy Choice)	11½-oz. meal	7.0	3.0	Tr.
(Stouffer's):				
Regular, & gravy	9⅞-oz. meal	14.0		
Lean Cuisine	9½-oz. meal	15.0		
(Weight Watchers) beef, Romana	8¾-oz. meal	13.0	4.0	9.0

FOOD DESCRIPTION	MEASURE OR QUANTITY	FATS IN GRAMS		
		Total	Saturated	Unsaturated
SALMON:				
Atlantic (USDA):				
Raw, meat only	4 oz.	15.2		
Canned, solids & liq., including bones	4 oz.	13.8		
Chinook or King (USDA):				
Raw, meat only	4 oz.	17.7	6.0	12.0
Canned, solids & liq., including bones, no salt added	4 oz.	15.9	4.0	11.0
Chum (USDA) canned, solids & liq., including bones, no salt added	4 oz.	5.9		
Coho (USDA) canned, solids & liq., no salt added	4 oz.	8.1		
Pink or Humpback (USDA):				
Raw, meat only	4 oz.	4.2	1.0	3.0
Raw, meat only, dipped in brine	4 oz.	4.2	1.0	3.0
Canned, solids & liq.:				
(USDA) no salt added	4 oz.	6.7	2.0	4.0
(Del Monte)	7¾-oz. can	9.2		
Sockeye or Red or Blueback, canned, solids & liq.:				
(USDA)	4 oz.	10.5		
(Del Monte)	7¾-oz. can	16.7		
Unspecified kind of salmon, baked or broiled with vegetable shortening (USDA)	4-oz. steak (approx. 4″ × 3″ × ½″, 4.2 oz.)	8.9		
SALMON, SMOKED:				
(USDA)	4 oz.	10.5		
Lox, drained (Vita)	4-oz. jar	6.7		
Nova, drained (Vita)	5-oz. can	14.6		
SALSIFY (USDA):				
Raw, without tops, freshly harvested	1 lb. (weighed untrimmed)	2.4		
Boiled, drained, freshly harvested or after storage	4 oz.	.7		
SALT:				
Butter-flavored, imitation:				
(Durkee)	1 tsp (5 grams)	.3		
(French's)	1 tsp. (4 grams)	.9		
Garlic (French's)	1 tsp. (6 grams)	.1		
Hickory smoke (French's)	1 tsp. (4 grams)	Tr.		
Onion (Lawry's)	1 tsp. (3 grams)	Tr.		
Substitute (Morton)	1 tsp (6 grams)	0.0		
Table (Morton) regular or lite	1 tsp. (6 grams)	0.0		
SALT PORK, raw (USDA):				
With skin	1 lb. (weighed with skin)	370.0	141.0	229.0
Without skin	1 oz.	24.1	9.0	15.0
SANDWICH SPREAD:				
(USDA) low-calorie	1 T. (.5 oz.)	1.4		
(Hellmann's)	1 T. (.5 oz.)	6.2		
(Oscar Mayer)	1 oz.	5.9	1.8	3.0
SAPODILLA, fresh (USDA) flesh only	4 oz.	1.2		
SAPOTE OR MARMALADE PLUM, fresh (USDA) flesh only	4 oz.	.7		
SARDINE:				
Atlantic, canned in oil (USDA):				
Solids & liq.	3¾-oz. can	25.9		
Drained solids	3¾-oz. can	10.2		
Atlantic, canned in tomato sauce, solids & liq. (Del Monte)	1½ large sardines	6.8		
Norwegian, canned:				
(Snow's)	1 oz.	6.3		
(Underwood):				
In mustard sauce	3¾-oz. can	14.2		

FOOD DESCRIPTION	MEASURE OR QUANTITY	FATS IN GRAMS		
		Total	Saturated	Unsaturated
In oil, drained	3¾-oz. can	16.0		
In tomato sauce	3¾-oz. can	9.8		
Pacific (USDA):				
Raw	4 oz.	9.8		
Canned, solids & liq.:				
In brine or mustard	4 oz.	13.6		
In tomato sauce	4 oz.	13.8		
SAUCE:				
Regular:				
A-1	1 T.	Tr.		
Barbecue:				
Chris' & Pitt's	1 T.	.1		
(Hunt's) any flavor	1 T.	Tr.		
Burrito (Del Monte)	¼ cup	0.0		
Caramel (Knorr)	1 T. (.7 oz.)	0.0		
Chili (See **CHILI SAUCE**)				
Grilling & broiling (Knorr):				
Chardonnay or tuscan herb	⅛ of container	4.0		
Spicy plum	⅛ of container	2.0		
Tequila lime	⅛ of container	2.9		
Hollandaise (Knorr) microwave	1/12 of container	5.0		
Hot (Gebhardt) Louisiana-style	1 tsp.	0.0		
Hot dog, *Just Right*	2 oz.	Tr.		
Italian (See also **SPAGHETTI SAUCE** or **TOMATO SAUCE**):				
(Contadina)	4-oz. serving	2.4		
(Ragú) red cooking	3½-oz. serving	2.0		
Mandarin ginger (Knorr) microwave	⅛ of container	3.6		
Newberg (Snow's) with sherry	⅓ cup	8.0		
Orange (La Choy) mandarin	1 T.	Tr.		
Parmesano (Knorr) microwave	⅛ of container	3.7		
Picante (Old El Paso)	1 T.	Tr.		
Plum (La Choy) tangy	1 oz.	.1		
Salsa brava (La Victoria)	1 T.	Tr.		
Salsa Jalapeña (La Victoria) green or red	1 T.	Tr.		
Salsa Mexicana (Contadina)	4 fl. oz.	.4		
Salsa Picante (Del Monte) regular	¼ cup	0.0		
Salsa Roja (Del Monte)	¼ cup	0.0		
Salsa Suprema (La Victoria)	1 T.	Tr.		
Salsa Victoria (La Victoria)	1 T.	Tr.		
Seafood cocktail (Del Monte)	1 T.	Tr.		
Soy (Kikkoman) or (La Choy)	1 T.	Tr.		
Sweet & sour (Chun King) or (La Choy)	1-oz. serving	Tr.		
Szechuan (La Choy) hot & spicy	1 oz.	.2		
Tabasco	¼ tsp.	Tr.		
Taco:				
(La Victoria) green or red	1 T.	Tr.		
(Ortega) hot	1 oz.	.1		
Tartar (Hellmann's)	1 T.	7.9	1.3	6.8
Teriyaki (Kikkoman)	1 T.	Tr.		
White, medium (USDA)	¼ cup	7.9	4.4	3.5
Worcestershire (French's) regular or smoky	1 T.	0.0		
Dietetic:				
Barbecue (Estee)	1 T.	0.0		

FOOD DESCRIPTION	MEASURE OR QUANTITY	FATS IN GRAMS		
		Total	Saturated	Unsaturated
Mexican (Pritikin)	1 oz.	Tr.		
Soy:				
(Kikkoman) lite	1 T.	Tr.		
(La Choy)	1 T.	0.0		
Steak (Estee)	.5 oz.	0.0		
Tartar (USDA)	1 T.	3.1		
SAUCE MIX:				
Regular:				
A la King (Durkee)	1-oz. pkg.	8.0		
*Au jus (Knorr)	2 fl. oz.	.2		
*Bernaise (Knorr)	2 fl. oz.	17.0		
*Cheese:				
(Durkee)	½ cup	10.5		
(French's)	½ cup	4.0		
*Demi-glace (Knorr)	2 fl. oz.	1.0		
Hollandaise:				
(Durkee)	1-oz. pkg.	14.0		
*(French's)	1 T.	1.3		
*(Knorr)	2 fl. oz.	18.0		
*Hunter (Knorr)	2 fl. oz.	.6		
*Italian (Knorr) Napoli	4 fl. oz.	3.0		
*Lyonnaise (Knorr)	2 fl. oz.	.4		
*Mushroom (Knorr)	2 fl. oz.	3.0		
*Pepper (Knorr)	2 fl. oz.	.6		
*Sour cream (French's)	⅔ cup	7.0		
*Sweet & sour (Kikkoman)	1 T.	0.0		
Teriyaki (Kikkoman)	1.5-oz. pkg.	.4		
Dietetic (Weight Watchers) lemon butter	1 pkg.	0.0		
SAUERKRAUT, canned:				
(USDA):				
Solids & liq., 1.9% salt	1 cup (8.3 oz.)	.5		
Drained solids	1 cup (5 oz.)	.4		
(Stokely-Van Camp's)	1 cup (7.8 oz.)	.4		
SAUSAGE:				
Brown & serve:				
*(USDA)	1 oz.	10.7		
*(Hormel)	1 sausage	6.5		
Country-style, smoked links				
(USDA)	1 oz.	8.8	3.1	5.7
Patty (Hormel) hot or mild	1 patty	13.0		
Polish-style:				
(Eckrich) meat:				
Regular	1 oz.	9.0		
Skinless	1 oz.	8.0		
(Hormel):				
Regular	1 sausage	7.0		
Kielbasa	½ link	14.0		
Kolbase	3 oz.	19.0		
Pork:				
(Eckrich):				
Links	1-oz. link	10.0		
Patty	2-oz. patty	26.0		
*(Hormel):				
Little Sizzlers	1 sausage	4.5		
Smoked	1 oz.	9.0		
(Jimmy Dean)	2 oz.	9.0		
*(Oscar Mayer) *Little Friers*	1-oz. link	6.8	2.4	4.0
Smoked:				
(Eckrich):				
Beef	2 oz.	17.0		
Cheese	2 oz.	15.0		
Ham, *Smok-Y-Links*	.8-oz. link	6.5		
Meat	2 oz.	17.0		
(Hormel) Smokies, regular or cheese	1 sausage	7.5		
(Oscar Mayer):				
Regular	1.5-oz. link	11.2		
Beef or cheese	1.5-oz. link	11.0		
Pork, Little Smokies	.3-oz. link	2.5		

FOOD DESCRIPTION	MEASURE OR QUANTITY	FATS IN GRAMS		
		Total	Saturated	Unsaturated
Turkey:				
*(Louis Rich)	1 oz.	3.0		
(Ohse) breakfast	1 oz.	5.3		
Vienna, canned (Libby's):				
In barbecue sauce	½ of 5-oz. can	15.0		
In beef broth	1 link (5-oz. can)	4.3		
SAUTERNES	Any quantity	0.0		
SCALLION (See **ONION, GREEN**)				
SCALLOP:				
Raw (USDA) muscle only	4 oz.	.2		
Steamed (USDA)	4 oz.	1.6		
Frozen:				
(USDA) breaded, fried, re-heated	4 oz.	9.5		
(Mrs. Paul's) breaded & french fried	½ of 7-oz. pkg.	7.0		
SCALLOP & SHRIMP MARINER, frozen (Stouffer's) with rice	10¼-oz. pkg.	16		
SCOTCH WHISKEY (See **DISTILLED LIQUOR**)				
SCRAPPLE (USDA)	4 oz.	15.4		
SCROD, frozen (Gorton's) microwave entree, baked	1 pkt.	18.0	4.0	14.0
SEABASS, WHITE, raw, meat only (USDA)	4 oz.	.6		
SEAFOOD DINNER OR ENTREE, frozen:				
(Armour) *Classics Lite,* natural herbs	10-oz. pkg.	2.0		
(Healthy Choice)	8-oz. meal	3.0	1.0	Tr.
SEGO DIET FOOD, canned:				
Regular:				
Very chocolate, very chocolate malt or very dutch chocolate	10-fl.-oz. can	1.0		
Very strawberry or very vanilla	10-fl.-oz. can	5.0		
Lite:				
Chocolate, chocolate jamocha almond, chocolate malt, double chocolate or dutch chocolate	10-fl.-oz. can	3.0		
French vanilla, strawberry or vanilla	10-fl.-oz. can	4.0		
SESAME SEED, dry (USDA) hulled	1 oz.	15.1	2.0	13.0
SHAD (USDA):				
Raw, meat only	4 oz.	11.3		
Cooked, home recipe:				
Baked with butter or margarine & bacon slices	4 oz.	12.8		
Creole, made with tomatoes, onion, green pepper, butter & flour	4 oz.	9.9		
Canned, solids & liq.	4 oz.	10.0		
SHAD, GIZZARD, raw (USDA) meat only	4 oz.	15.9		
SHAKE 'n BAKE, seasoned mixes:				
Chicken:				
Original recipe	5½-oz. pkg.	14.0		
Barbecue	7-oz. pkg.	16.4		
Italian herb	5¾-oz. pkg.	11.1		
Fish, original recipe	5¼-oz. pkg.	10.5		
Pork or ribs:				
Original recipe	6-oz. pkg.	8.7		
Barbecue	5¾-oz. pkg.	13.7		

FOOD DESCRIPTION	MEASURE OR QUANTITY	FATS IN GRAMS		
		Total	Saturated	Unsaturated
SHAKEY'S:				
Chicken, fried, & potatoes:				
3-piece	1 order	56.0		
5-piece	1 order	90.0		
Ham & cheese sandwich, hot	1 sandwich	21.0		
Pizza:				
Cheese, thick	13" pizza	43.0		
Onion, green pepper, olive & mushroom, thin	13" pizza	54.0		
Pepperoni, thick	13" pizza	81.0		
Sausage & mushroom, thin	13" pizza	58.0		
Sausage & pepperoni, thin	13" pizza	102.0		
Special, thick	13" pizza	96.0		
Potatoes	15-piece order	36.0		
Spaghetti with meat sauce & garlic bread	1 order	33.0		
Super hot hero	1 sandwich	44.0		
SHALLOT, raw (USDA) with or without skin	1 oz.	Tr.		
SHEEPSHEAD, Atlantic, raw (USDA) meat only	4 oz.	3.2		
SHELLS, PASTA, STUFFED, frozen:				
(Buitoni) jumbo:				
Cheese	5½-oz. serving	13.7	8.5	4.3
Florentine	5½-oz. serving	12.5	7.8	3.8
(Celentano):				
Broccoli & cheese stuffed	11¼-oz. pkg. (4 shells)	17.0		
Cheese stuffed, with sauce	½ of 16-oz. box	14.0		
SHERBET OR SORBET:				
Lemon (Häagen-Dazs)	4 fl. oz.	Tr.		
Orange:				
(Baskin-Robbins)	4 fl. oz.	2.4		
(Dole) mandarin	½ cup	Tr.		
Peach (Dole)	½ cup	Tr.		
Pineapple (Dole)	½ cup	Tr.		
Rainbow (Baskin-Robbins)	1 scoop (4 fl. oz.)	2.0		
Raspberry:				
(Baskin-Robbins)	4 fl. oz.	0.0		
(Häagen-Dazs)	4 fl. oz.	Tr.		
SHERBET OR SORBET & ICE CREAM (Häagen-Dazs):				
Bar, orange & cream	2.6-fl.-oz. bar	6.0		
Bulk:				
Blueberry & cream, orange & cream, or raspberry & cream	4 fl. oz.	8.0		
Key lime & cream	4 fl. oz.	7.0		
SHERBET SHAKE, mix (Weight Watchers) orange	1 envelope	0.0		
SHERRY	Any quantity	0.0		
SHORTENING (See **FATS**)				
SHREDDED OATS, cereal (USDA)	1 oz.	6.0	Tr.	<1.0
SHREDDED WHEAT, cereal:	1 cup (1.2 oz.)	2.0		
(Kellogg's) cinnamon or sugar-frosted, *Mini-Wheats*	4 biscuits (1 oz.)	.3		
(Nabisco):				
Regular	1 biscuit (.9 oz.)	1.0		
Spoon Size	⅔ cup (1 oz.)	1.0		
SHRIMP:				
Raw (USDA):				
Whole	1 lb. (weighed in shell)	2.5		
Meat only	4 oz.	.9		
Cooked, french-fried, dipped in egg, bread crumbs & flour or in batter (USDA)	4 oz.	12.2		
Canned, dry pack or drained (USDA)	1 cup (22 large or 76 small, 4.5 oz.)	1.4		

FOOD DESCRIPTION	MEASURE OR QUANTITY	FATS IN GRAMS		
		Total	Saturated	Unsaturated
SHRIMP COCKTAIL (Sau-Sea)	4-oz. jar	1.0		
SHRIMP, DINNER OR ENTREE, frozen:				
(Armour) *Classics Lite:*				
Baby bay	9¾-oz. meal	6.0		
Creole	11¼-oz. meal	2.0		
(Gorton's):				
Crunchy whole	5-oz. serving	20.0	3.0	17.0
Scampi, microwave	1 package	32.0	14.0	18.0
(Healthy Choice) creole or marinara	1 meal	1.0	Tr.	Tr.
(La choy) Fresh & Lite, with lobster sauce	10-oz. meal	6.2		
(Stouffer's) *Right Course,* primavera	9⅝-oz. meal	7.0		
SHRIMP PASTE, canned (USDA)	1 oz.	2.7		
SKATE, raw (USDA) meat only	4 oz.	.8		
***SLOPPY JOE SEASONING MIX:**				
(Durkee):				
Regular	1¼ cups	48.5		
Pizza flavor	1¼ cups	51.0		
(Hunt's) *Manwich*	5.9-oz. serving	13.0		
SMELT, Atlantic, jack & bay (USDA) canned, solids & liq.	4 oz.	15.3		
SNAIL, raw (USDA)	4 oz.	1.6		
SNAPPER (See **RED SNAPPER**)				
SOFT DRINK:				
Carbonated, regular or dietetic, any flavor	Any quantity	0.0		
Chocolate (Yoo-Hoo)	6 fl. oz.	.7		
SOLE:				
Raw (USDA) meat only	4 oz.	.9		
Frozen:				
(Frionor) *Norway Gourmet*	4-oz. fillet	0.0		
(Gorton's):				
Fishmarket Fresh	4 oz.	1.0		
Microwave entree, with lemon butter sauce	1 pkg.	24.0	11.0	13.0
(Healthy Choice):				
Dinner, au gratin	11-oz. meal	5.0	3.0	Tr.
Entree, with lemon butter sauce	8¼-oz. meal	4.0	2.0	1.0
(Weight Watchers) stuffed, with Newburg sauce	10½-oz. meal	9.0	1.0	8.0
SORGHUM (USDA) grain	1 oz.	.9	Tr.	Tr.
SOUFFLÉ:				
Cheese, home recipe (USDA)	4 oz.	19.4	10.0	9.2
Corn, frozen (Stouffer's)	4 oz.	7.0		
Spinach, frozen (Stouffer's)	4 oz.	9.0		
SOUP:				
Canned, regular pack:				
*Asparagus (Campbell), condensed:				
Cream of	8-oz. serving	4.0		
Creamy Natural	8-oz. serving	14.0		
Bean:				
(Campbell's):				
Chunky, with ham, old-fashioned	11-oz. can	9.0		
*Condensed, with bacon	8-oz. serving	5.0		
*Semi-condensed, *Soup For One,* with ham	11-oz. serving	7.0		
(Grandma Brown's)	8-oz. serving	3.4		
Bean, black:				
*(Campbell's) condensed	8-oz. serving	2.0		
(Crosse & Blackwell) with sherry	6½-oz. serving	1.0		

FOOD DESCRIPTION	MEASURE OR QUANTITY	FATS IN GRAMS		
		Total	Saturated	Unsaturated
Beef:				
(Campbell's):				
Chunky:				
Regular	10¾-oz. can	5.0		
Stroganoff style	10¾-oz. can	15.0		
*Condensed:				
Regular	8-oz. serving	2.0		
Broth or consommé	8-oz. serving	0.0		
Mushroom	8-oz. serving	3.0		
Noodle:				
Regular	8-oz. serving	3.0		
Homestyle	8-oz. serving	4.0		
(Progresso):				
Regular	10½-oz. can	7.0		
Noodle	½ of 19-oz. can	4.0		
Tomato, with rotini	½ of 19-oz. can	6.0		
Vegetable	½ of 19-oz. can	3.0		
(Swanson)	7¼-oz. can	1.0		
Beef barley (Progresso)	10½-oz. can	5.0		
Borscht (See **BORSCHT**)				
*Broccoli (Campbell's) condensed, _Creamy Natural_	8-oz. serving	8.0		
*Cauliflower (Campbell's) condensed, _Creamy Natural_	8-oz. serving	13.0		
Celery:				
*(Campbell's) condensed, cream of	8-oz. serving	7.0		
*(Rokeach):				
Prepared with milk	10-oz. serving	9.0		
Prepared with water	10-oz. serving	4.0		
Chickarina (Progresso)	½ of 19-oz. can	5.0		
Chicken:				
(Campbell's):				
Chunky:				
Noodle, with mushrooms	10¾-oz. can	7.0		
Old-fashioned	10¾-oz. can	5.0		
With rice	19-oz. can	8.0		
Vegetable	19-oz. can	12.0		
*Condensed:				
Alphabet	8-oz. serving	3.0		
Broth:				
Plain or noodle	8-oz. serving	2.0		
& rice	8-oz. serving	1.0		
Cream of	8-oz. serving	7.0		
Mushroom, creamy	8-oz. serving	8.0		
Noodle	8-oz. serving	3.0		
& rice	8-oz. serving	2.0		
Vegetable	8-oz. serving	3.0		
*Semi-condensed, _Soup-For One:_				
& noodles, golden	11-oz. serving	4.0		
Vegetable, full-flavored	11-oz. serving	6.0		
(Hain):				
Broth	8¾-oz. serving	6.0		
Noodle	9½-oz. serving	4.0		
(Progresso):				
Barley	½ of 18½-oz. serving	2.0		
Broth	4 oz.	0.0		
Cream of	½ of 19-oz. can	11.0		
Hearty, noodle, rice or vegetable	10½-oz. can	4.0		
(Swanson) broth	7¼-oz. can	2.0		
Chowder:				
Beef'n vegetable (Hormel) _Short Orders_	7½-oz. can	5.0		

FOOD DESCRIPTION	MEASURE OR QUANTITY	FATS IN GRAMS		
		Total	Saturated	Unsaturated
Clam:				
Manhattan-style:				
(Campbell's):				
Chunky:				
Small	10¾-oz. can	5.0		
Large	19-oz. can	8.0		
*Condensed	8-oz. serving	2.0		
(Crosse & Blackwell)	6½-oz. serving	1.0		
(Progresso)	½ of 19-oz. can	2.0		
New England-style:				
(Campbell's):				
Chunky	10¾-oz. can	17.0		
*Condensed:				
Made with milk	8-oz. serving	7.0		
Made with water	8-oz. serving	3.0		
*Semi-condensed,				
Soup For One:				
Made with milk	11-oz. serving	8.0		
Made with water	11-oz. serving	4.0		
(Crosse & Blackwell)	6½-oz. serving	3.0		
(Progresso)	10½-oz. can	13.0		
*(Snow's) made with milk	7½-oz. serving	6.0		
Corn:				
(Progresso)	½ of 18½-oz. can	10.0		
*(Snow's) condensed, made with milk	7½-oz. serving	6.0		
*Fish (Snow's) condensed, made with milk	7½-oz. serving	6.0		
Consommé madrilene (Crosse & Blackwell)	6½-oz. serving	2.0		
Crab (Crosse & Blackwell)	6½-oz. serving	1.0		
Escarole (Progresso) in chicken broth	½ of 18½-oz. can	1.0		
Gazpacho:				
*(Campbell's) condensed	8-oz. serving	0.0		
(Crosse & Blackwell)	6½-oz. serving	2.0		
Ham'n butter bean (Campbell's) *Chunky*	10¾-oz. can	10.0		
Lentil:				
(Hain) vegetarian	9½-oz. serving	3.0		
(Progresso):				
Regular	10½-oz. serving	4.0		
With sausage	½ of 19-oz. can	7.0		
Macaroni & bean (Progresso)	10½-oz. can	4.0		
Minestrone:				
(Campbell's):				
Chunky	19-oz. can	10.0		
*Condensed	8-oz. serving	2.0		
(Crosse & Blackwell)	6½-oz. serving	2.0		
(Hain)	9½-oz. serving	2.0		
(Progresso):				
Beef	10½-oz. can	5.0		
Hearty	½ of 18½-oz. can	2.0		
Zesty	½ of 19-oz. can	8.0		
Mushroom:				
*(Campbell's) condensed:				
Cream of	8-oz. serving	7.0		
Golden	8-oz. serving	3.0		
(Crosse & Blackwell) cream of, bisque	6½-oz. serving	5.0		
(Hain) creamy	9¼-oz. serving	4.0		
(Progresso) cream of	½ of 18½-oz. can	10.0		
*(Rokeach) cream of, prepared with water	10-oz. serving	10.0		
Mushroom barley (Hain)	9½-oz. serving	2.0		
*Noodle (Campbell's):				
Curly, & chicken	8-oz. serving	3.0		
& ground beef	8-oz. serving	4.0		

FOOD DESCRIPTION	MEASURE OR QUANTITY	FATS IN GRAMS		
		Total	Saturated	Unsaturated
*Onion (Campbell's):				
Regular	8-oz. serving	2.0		
Cream of:				
Made with water	8-oz. serving	5.0		
Made with milk &				
water	8-oz. serving	7.0		
*Pea, green (Campbell's)				
condensed	8-oz. serving	3.0		
Pea, split:				
(Campbell's):				
Chunky, with ham	10¾-oz. can	6.0		
*Condensed, with ham				
& bacon	8-oz. serving	4.0		
(Grandma Brown's)	8-oz. serving	3.0		
(Progresso):				
Regular	10½-oz. can	3.0		
With ham	10½-oz. can	4.0		
*Potato (Campbell's):				
Condensed, cream of:				
Made with water	8-oz. serving	3.0		
Made with milk &				
water	8-oz. serving	4.0		
Creamy Natural	8-oz. serving	15.0		
*Scotch broth (Campbell's)				
condensed	8-oz. serving	3.0		
Shav (Manischewitz)	1 cup	Tr.	0.0	Tr.
Shrimp:				
*(Campbell's) condensed,				
cream of:				
Made with milk	8-oz. serving	10.0		
Made with water	8-oz. serving	6.0		
(Crosse & Blackwell)	6½-oz. serving	4.0		
Sirloin burger (Campbell's)				
Chunky	19-oz. can	16.0		
*Spinach (Campbell's)				
condensed, *Creamy*				
Natural	8-oz. serving	10.0		
Steak & potato (Campbell's)				
Chunky	19-oz. can	8.0		
Tomato:				
(Campbell's):				
*Condensed:				
Regular:				
Made with milk	8-oz. serving	6.0		
Made with water	8-oz. serving	2.0		
Creamy Natural	8-oz. serving	7.0		
& rice, old-fashioned	8-oz. serving	2.0		
*Semi-condensed, *Soup*				
For One, Royale	11-oz. serving	3.0		
*(Rokeach):				
Plain, made with water	10-oz. serving	1.0		
& rice	10-oz. serving	5.0		
Tortellini (Progresso):				
Regular	½ of 19-oz. can	3.0		
Creamy	½ of 18½-oz. can	16.0		
Turkey (Campbell's):				
Chunky	18¾-oz. can	12.0		
*Condensed:				
Noodle	8-oz. serving	2.0		
Vegetable	8-oz. serving	3.0		
Vegetable:				
(Campbell's):				
Chunky:				
Regular	10¾-oz. can	4.0		
Beef, old-fashioned:				
Small	10¾-oz. can	5.0		
Large	19-oz. can	8.0		
*Condensed, regular,				
beef, old-fashioned				
or vegetarian	8-oz. serving	2.0		

FOOD DESCRIPTION	MEASURE OR QUANTITY	FATS IN GRAMS		
		Total	Saturated	Unsaturated
*Semi-condensed, *Soup For One:*				
Barley, with beef & bacon	11-oz. serving	5.0		
Old world	11-oz. serving	4.0		
(Hain):				
Broth	9½-oz. serving	0.0		
Chicken or vegetarian	9½-oz. serving	4.0		
(Progresso)	10½-oz. serving	2.0		
*(Rokeach) vegetarian	10-oz. serving	3.0		
Vichyssoise (Crosse & Blackwell) cream of	6½-oz. serving	4.0		
*Won ton (Campbell's)	8-oz. serving	1.0		
Canned, dietetic pack:				
Beef (Campbell) *Chunky,* & mushroom, low-sodium	10¾-oz. can	7.0		
Chicken:				
(Campbell's) low-sodium, & vegetable	10¾-oz. can	11.0		
(Estee) & vegetable	7¼-oz. serving	7.0		
(Hain) low-sodium:				
Broth	8¾-oz. serving	5.0		
Noodle	9½-oz. serving	4.0		
(Pritikin):				
Broth, defatted	½ of 13¾-oz. can	0.0		
Gumbo	½ of 14¾-oz. can	1.0		
(Weight Watchers) noodle	10½-oz. can	2.0		
Chowder, clam (Pritikin) Manhattan or New England style	½ of 14¾-oz. can	Tr.		
Italian vegetable pasta (Hain) low-sodium	9½-oz. serving	6.0		
Lentil:				
(Hain) vegetarian	9½-oz. serving	3.0		
(Pritikin)	½ of 14¾-oz. can	0.0		
Minestrone:				
(Estee) chunky	7½-oz. serving	8.0		
(Hain)	9½-oz. serving	4.0		
(Pritikin)	½ of 14¾-oz. can	Tr.		
Mushroom:				
(Campbell's) cream of, low-sodium	10½-oz. can	14.0		
(Weight Watchers)	10½-oz. can	2.0		
Onion (Campbell's) French, low-sodium	10½-oz. can	5.0		
Pea, split (Campbell's) low-sodium	10¾-oz. can	5.0		
Tomato (Campbell's) low-sodium, with tomato pieces	10½-oz. can	5.0		
Turkey:				
(Hain) & rice	9½-oz. serving	3.0		
(Pritikin) vegetable, with ribbon pasta	½ of 14¾-oz. can	Tr.		
(Weight Watchers) vegetable	10½-oz. can	2.0		
Vegetable:				
(Campbell) low-sodium, *Chunky*	10¾-oz. can	5.0		
(Estee) & beef	7½-oz. serving	7.0		
(Hain) low-sodium:				
Broth	9½-oz. serving	Tr.		
Vegetarian	9½-oz. serving	5.0		
(Pritikin)	½ of 14¾-oz. can	0.0		
(Weight Watchers) with beef stock or vegetarian, chunky	10½-oz. can	2.0		
Frozen:				
Asparagus (Kettle Ready) cream of	6 oz.	4.3		

FOOD DESCRIPTION	MEASURE OR QUANTITY	FATS IN GRAMS		
		Total	Saturated	Unsaturated
Barley & mushroom:				
(Empire Kosher)	½ of 15-oz. polybag	0.0		
(Tabatchnick)	8 oz.	2.0		
Bean (Kettle Ready) with ham:				
Black	6 oz.	6.2		
Savory	6 oz.	3.6	1.0	2.4
Bean & barley				
(Tabatchnick)	8 oz.	2.0		
Beef (Kettle Ready) vegetable	6 oz.	2.8	.6	1.8
Broccoli, cream of:				
(Kettle Ready):				
Regular	6 oz.	7.2	2.6	3.4
Cheddar	6 oz.	11.3	5.2	4.7
(Tabatchnick)	7½ oz.	4.0		
Cauliflower (Kettle Ready) cream of	6 oz.	6.9	3.1	3.0
Cheese (Kettle Ready) cream of, cheddar	6 oz.	12.5	6.1	5.7
Chicken:				
(Empire Kosher) noodle	½ of 15-oz. polybag	2.0		
(Kettle Ready):				
Cream of	6 oz.	6.2	2.3	3.2
Gumbo	6 oz.	3.5	.7	2.4
Noodle	6 oz.	2.9	.6	1.8
Chili (Kettle Ready) jalapeño	6 oz.	7.8	2.1	4.9
Chowder:				
Clam:				
Boston (Kettle Ready)	6 oz.	7.3	1.5	4.7
Manhattan:				
(Kettle Ready)	6 oz.	2.6	.5	1.8
(Tabatchnick)	7½ oz.	1.5		
New England (Kettle Ready)	6 oz.	6.5	2.4	3.2
Corn & broccoli (Kettle Ready)	6 oz.	5.0	1.8	2.5
Lentil (Tabatchnick)	8 oz.	2.0		
Minestrone:				
(Kettle Ready)	6 oz.	4.4	1.1	2.5
(Tabatchnick)	8 oz.	2.0		
Mushroom (Kettle Ready) cream of	6 oz.	6.4	2.4	3.1
Onion (Kettle Ready)	6 oz.	2.2	.4	1.6
Pea:				
(Empire Kosher)	½ of 15-oz. polybag	0.0		
(Tabatchnick)	8 oz.	2.0		
Pea, split (Kettle Ready)	6 oz.	4.4	1.3	2.8
Potato (Tabatchnick)	8 oz.	1.0		
Spinach (Stouffer's) cream of	8 oz.	15.0		
Tomato (Empire Kosher) & rice	½ of 15-oz. polybag	1.0		
Turkey chili (Empire Kosher)	½ of 15-oz. polybag	12.0		
Vegetable:				
(Empire Kosher)	½ of 15-oz. polybag	Tr.		
(Kettle Ready) garden	6 oz.	2.8	.5	1.8
*Won Ton (La Choy)	½ of 15-oz. pkg.	1.0		
Mix, regular:				
*Asparagus (Knorr)	8 oz.	3.0		
*Barley (Knorr) country	10 oz.	1.8		
Beef:				
*Carmel Kosher	6 oz.	.1		
*(Lipton) Cup-A-Soup:				
Regular:				
Noodle	6 fl. oz.	.7		
Vegetable	6 fl. oz.	Tr.		
Lots-A-Noodles	7 fl. oz.	1.3		

FOOD DESCRIPTION	MEASURE OR QUANTITY	FATS IN GRAMS		
		Total	Saturated	Unsaturated
*Broccoli (Lipton) creamy, *Cup-A-Soup:*				
Regular	6 fl. oz.	2.4		
& cheese	6 fl. oz.	3.4		
*Cauliflower (Knorr)	8 oz.	3.0		
*Cheese (Hain) savory	3/4 cup	16.0		
*Cheese & broccoli (Hain)	3/4 cup	22.0		
*Chicken:				
(Knorr)	8 oz.	1.5		
(Lipton):				
Regular, noodle	8 fl. oz.	Tr.		
Cup-A-Broth	6 fl. oz.	Tr.		
Cup-A-Soup:				
Regular:				
Cream of	6 fl. oz.	4.0		
& noodles with				
meat	6 fl. oz.	1.0		
& rice	6 fl. oz.	Tr.		
Country-style:				
Hearty	6 fl. oz.	1.0		
Supreme	6 fl. oz.	5.0		
Lots-A-Noodles:				
Regular	7 fl. oz.	1.0		
Cream of	7 fl. oz.	5.0		
*Chowder (Gorton's) New England	1/4 of pkg.	5.0		
*Herb (Knorr) fine	8 oz.	6.0		
*Hot & sour (Knorr) oriental	8 oz.	3.0		
*Leek (Knorr)	8 oz.	4.0		
*Lentil (Hain)	3/4 cup	2.0		
*Minestrone:				
(Knorr)	10 oz.	2.0		
(Manischewitz)	6 oz.	Tr.		
*Mushroom:				
(Hain)	3/4 cup	15.0		
(Knorr)	8 oz.	4.0		
(Lipton):				
Regular, beef	8 fl. oz.	Tr.		
Cup-A-Soup, cream of	6 fl. oz.	4.0		
*Noodle (Lipton):				
With chicken broth	8 fl. oz.	2.0		
Ring-O-Noodle	8 fl. oz.	1.0		
*Onion:				
(Hain)	3/4 cup	2.0		
(Knorr) French	8 oz.	.8		
(Lipton):				
Regular:				
Plain	8 fl. oz.	Tr.		
Beefy	8 fl. oz.	1.0		
Cup-A-Soup	6 fl. oz.	1.0		
*Oxtail (Knorr) hearty beef	8 oz.	2.3		
*Pea, green (Lipton) *Cup-A-Soup:*				
Regular, green	6 fl. oz.	4.0		
Country-style, Virginia	6 fl. oz.	5.0		
*Pea, split (Manischewitz)	6 fl. oz.	Tr.		
*Potato leek (Hain)	3/4 cup	18.0		
*Tomato:				
(Hain)	3/4 cup	14.0		
(Knorr) basil	8 oz.	2.6		
*Tortellini (Knorr) in brodo	8 oz.	1.1		
*Vegetable:				
(Hain)	3/4 cup	1.0		
(Knorr) plain or spring with herbs	8 oz.	Tr.		
(Lipton):				
Regular:				
Beef stock	8 fl. oz.	Tr.		
For dip	8 fl. oz.	1.0		

FOOD DESCRIPTION	MEASURE OR QUANTITY	FATS IN GRAMS		
		Total	Saturated	Unsaturated
Cup-A-Soup:				
Regular:				
Beef	6 fl. oz.	Tr.		
Spring	6 fl. oz.	1.0		
Country-style, harvest	6 fl. oz.	Tr.		
(Manischewitz)	6 fl. oz.	Tr.		
*Mix, dietetic:				
Beef:				
(Estee) noodle	6 fl. oz.	Tr.		
(Weight Watchers) broth	6 fl. oz.	0.0		
Broccoli (Lipton) *Cup-A-Soup,* golden, lite	6 fl. oz.	1.2		
Chicken:				
(Estee) noodle	6 fl. oz.	Tr.		
(Weight Watchers) broth	6 fl. oz.	0.0		
Mushroom:				
(Estee) cream of	6 fl. oz.	2.0		
(Hain)	¾ cup	20.0		
Onion:				
(Estee)	6 fl. oz.	Tr.		
(Hain)	¾ cup	1.0		
SOURSOP, raw (USDA) flesh only	4 oz.	.3		
SOUTHERN COMFORT	1 fl. oz.	0.0		
SOYBEAN (USDA):				
Young seeds:				
Raw	1 lb. (weighed in pods)	12.3	2.0	10.0
Cooked without salt, drained	4 oz.	4.8	1.0	5.0
Canned:				
Solids & liq.	4 oz.	3.6	1.0	2.0
Drained solids	4 oz.	5.7	1.0	5.0
Mature seeds, dry:				
Raw	1 cup (7.4 oz.)	37.2	6.0	31.0
Cooked without salt	4 oz.	6.5	1.0	6.0
Roasted, *Soy Town,* with or without salt	1 oz.	10.5	1.0	9.0
SOYBEAN CURD OR TOFU (USDA)	4.2-oz. cake (2¾" × 2½")	5.0	1.0	4.0
SOYBEAN GRITS, high-fat (USDA)	1 cup (4.9 oz.)	16.7	3.0	14.0
SOYBEAN MILK (USDA):				
Fluid	4 oz.	1.7		
Powder	1 oz.	5.8	Tr.	5.0
Sweetened:				
Liquid concentrate	4 oz. (by wt.)	8.0	1.0	7.0
Dry powder	1 oz.	6.6	3.0	4.0
SOYBEAN PROTEIN (USDA)	1 oz.	Tr.		
SOYBEAN PROTEINATE (USDA)	1 oz.	Tr.		
SOYBEAN SPROUT (See **BEAN SPROUT**)				
SOYNUT, unsalted, *Soy Ahoy*	1 oz.	10.2	1.0	9.0
SOY SAUCE (See **SAUCE**)				
SPAGHETTI:				
Dry:				
(Mueller's)	1 oz.	.5		
(Pritikin) whole wheat	1 oz.	1.0		
Cooked (USDA):				
8–10 minutes	1 cup (5.1 oz.)	.7		
14–20 minutes	1 cup (4.9 oz.)	.6		
Canned:				
Regular:				
(Franco-American):				
Regular:				
With meatballs in tomato sauce or in meat sauce	1 can	8.0		

FOOD DESCRIPTION	MEASURE OR QUANTITY	FATS IN GRAMS		
		Total	Saturated	Unsaturated
SpaghettiOs:				
With meatballs	7⅜-oz. can	8.0		
With sliced franks	7⅜-oz. can	9.0		
(Hormel) & beef	7½-oz. can	14.0		
Dietetic (Estee) with meatballs	7½-oz. can	15.0		
Frozen:				
(Armour) *Dining Lite*	9-oz. meal	8.0		
(Banquet) casserole	8-oz. casserole	8.0		
(Healthy Choice)	10-oz. meal	6.0	2.0	2.0
(Kid Cuisine)	9¼-oz. meal	12.0		
(Stouffer's):				
Regular:				
With meatballs	12⅝-oz. meal	15.0		
With meat sauce	12⅞-oz. meal	11.0		
Lean Cuisine, with beef & mushroom sauce	11½-oz. meal	7.0		
(Weight Watchers) with meat sauce	10½-oz. meal	7.0	3.0	4.0
SPAGHETTI SAUCE, canned:				
Regular pack:				
Alfredo (Progresso) authentic pasta sauce:				
Regular	½ cup	30.0	1.0	19.0
Seafood	½ cup	19.0	12.0	1.0
Beef (Prego Plus)	4 oz.	7.0		
Bolognese (Progresso) authentic pasta sauce	½ cup	8.0	2.0	Tr.
Clam (Progresso):				
Red	½ cup	3.0		
White:				
Regular	½ cup	8.0		
Authentic pasta sauce	½ cup	9.0	1.0	Tr.
Homestyle:				
(Hunt's)	4 oz.	2.0		
(Ragú) plain, with mushrooms or meat flavor	4 oz.	2.0		
Lobster (Progresso) rock	½ cup	8.0	1.0	2.5
Marinara:				
(Progresso):				
Regular	½ cup	5.0	1.0	3.0
Authentic pasta sauce	½ cup	6.0	1.5	Tr.
(Ragú)	¼ of 15½-oz. can	4.0		
Meat:				
(Hunt's)	4 oz.	2.0		
(Progresso)	½ cup	5.0	1.0	2.0
(Ragú):				
Regular	4 oz.	2.0		
Extra Thick & Zesty	4 oz.	4.0		
Meatless or plain:				
(Prego)	4 oz.	6.0		
(Progresso)	½ cup	5.0	1.0	2.0
Mushroom:				
(Hunt's) homestyle	4 oz.	1.0		
(Progresso)	½ cup	5.0	1.0	2.0
Primavera (Progresso) creamy	½ cup	17.0	10.0	1.4
Sausage & green pepper (Prego Plus)	4 oz.	9.0		
Seafood (Progresso):				
Regular	½ cup	6.0	Tr.	Tr.
Authentic pasta sauce	½ cup	15.0	Tr.	9.0
Sicilian (Progresso)	½ cup	2.5	Tr.	Tr.
Traditional (Hunt's)	4 oz.	2.0		
Dietetic:				
(Estee)	4 oz.	1.0	Tr.	
(Pritikin) plain or mushroom	4 oz.	0.0		
(Weight Watchers) meat flavored	⅓ cup	1.0		

FOOD DESCRIPTION	MEASURE OR QUANTITY	FATS IN GRAMS		
		Total	Saturated	Unsaturated
*SPAGHETTI SAUCE MIX:				
(Durkee) plain	½ cup	.2		
(Spatini)	½ cup	0.0		
SPAM (Hormel) canned, regular or cheese	3 oz.	24.0		
SPANISH MACKEREL, raw				
(USDA) meat only	4 oz.	11.8		
SPARKLING COOLER CITRUS (La Croix) 3½% alcohol	12 fl. oz.	0.0		
SPECIAL K, cereal (Kellogg's)	1 cup (1 oz.)	0.0		
SPINACH:				
Raw (USDA):				
Trimmed or packaged	1 lb.	1.4		
Trimmed, chopped	1 cup (1.8 oz.)	Tr.		
Boiled, without salt (USDA) whole leaves, drained	1 cup (5.5 oz.)	.5		
Canned, regular pack: (USDA):				
Solids & liq.	½ cup (4.1 oz.)	.5		
Drained solids	½ cup (4 oz.)	.7		
(Stokely-Van Camp's) solids & liq.	½ cup (3.9 oz.)	.5		
Canned, dietetic pack, low-sodium:				
(USDA) solids & liq.	4 oz.	.5		
(Blue Boy) solids & liq.	4 oz.	.4		
Frozen:				
(Birds Eye):				
Chopped or leaf	⅓ of 10-oz. pkg.	.3		
Creamed	⅓ of 10-oz. pkg.	3.8		
(Green Giant):				
In butter sauce, cut leaf	½ of 10-oz. pkg.	2.0	Tr.	0.0
Creamed	⅓ of 10-oz. pkg.	1.7	1.0	Tr.
Harvest Fresh or polybag	4 oz.	0.0		
SPINACH, NEW ZEALAND (See **NEW ZEALAND SPINACH**)				
SPLEEN, raw (USDA):				
Beef & calf	4 oz.	3.4		
Hog or lamb	4 oz.	4.4		
SQUAB, pigeon, raw (USDA):				
Meat & skin	4 oz.	27.0		
Meat only	4 oz.	8.5		
Light meat only, without skin	4 oz.	4.8		
Giblets	1 oz.	2.0		
SQUASH SEEDS, dry (USDA) hulled	1 oz.	13.2	2.0	11.0
SQUASH, SUMMER:				
Fresh (USDA):				
Crookneck & Straightneck, yellow, boiled, drained, diced or sliced	½ cup	.2		
Scallop, white & pale green, boiled, drained, mashed	½ cup (4.2 oz.)	.1		
Zucchini & Cocazelle, green, boiled, drained slices	½ cup (4.1 oz.)	2.1		
Canned, zucchini:				
(Del Monte) in tomato sauce	½ cup (4.1 oz.)	.1		
(Progresso) Italian-style	½ cup	2.0	Tr.	Tr.
Frozen:				
(Birds Eye) summer squash or zucchini	3.3 oz.	.1		
(Ore-Ida) zucchini, breaded	3 oz.	9.0	2.0	7.0
SQUASH, WINTER:				
Fresh (USDA):				
Acorn, baked or boiled, flesh only, mashed	½ cup	.1		

FOOD DESCRIPTION	MEASURE OR QUANTITY	FATS IN GRAMS		
		Total	Saturated	Unsaturated
Butternut, baked or boiled, flesh only	4 oz.	.1		
Hubbard, baked, flesh only	4 oz.	.5		
Frozen:				
(USDA)	4 oz.	.3		
(Birds Eye)	⅓ of 12-oz. pkg.	.3		
SQUID, raw, meat only (USDA)	4 oz.	10.2		
STARCH (See **CORNSTARCH**)				
STOMACH, PORK, scalded (USDA)	4 oz.	10.2		
STRAWBERRY:				
Fresh (USDA):				
Whole	1 lb. (weighed with caps & stems)	2.2		
Whole, capped	1 cup (5.1 oz.)	.7		
Canned (USDA) unsweetened or low-calorie water pack, solids & liq.	4 oz.	.1		
Frozen:				
(USDA) sweetened:				
Whole	½ cup (4.5 oz.)	.3		
Sliced, not thawed	10-oz. pkg.	.6		
(Birds Eye) whole	¼ of 1-lb. pkg.	.2		
STRAWBERRY JELLY, sweetened (Home Brand)	1 T.	0.0		
STRAWBERRY PRESERVE OR JAM:				
Sweetened (Bama)	1 T. (.7 oz.)	0.0		
Dietetic or low-calorie (Estee)	1 T.	0.0		
STUFFING MIX:				
*Beef (Stove Top)	½ cup	8.7		
*Chicken:				
(Bell's)	½ cup	13.0		
*(Betty Crocker)	⅕ of pkg.	9.0		
Cornbread:				
(Pepperidge Farm)	⅛ of 8-oz. pkg.	1.0		
*(Stove Top)	½ cup	8.6		
*Herb (Betty Crocker)	⅙ of pkg.	9.0		
*Pork (Stove Top)	½ cup	8.9		
*Turkey (Stove Top)	½ cup	8.8		
STURGEON (USDA):				
Smoked	4 oz.	2.0		
Steamed	4 oz.	6.5		
SUCCOTASH, frozen (Birds Eye)	½ cup (3.3 oz.)	.5		
SUCKER, CARP, raw (USDA) meat only	4 oz.	3.6		
SUDDENLY SALAD (Betty Crocker):				
Caesar	⅙ of pkg.	8.0		
Classic pasta or Italian pasta	⅙ of pkg.	6.0		
Creamy macaroni	⅙ of pkg.	10.0		
SUET, raw (USDA)	1 oz.	26.6		
SUGAR, beet or cane (USDA)	Any quantity	0.0		
SUGAR APPLE, raw (USDA) flesh only	4 oz.	.3		
SUGAR FROSTED FLAKES, cereal (Kellogg's)	¾ cup (1 oz.)	0.0		
SUGAR PUFFS, cereal (Malt-O-Meal)	1 cup (1 oz.)	.4		
SUGAR SUBSTITUTE, any brand, any type	Any quantity	0.0		
SUNFLOWER SEED (USDA) hulled	1 oz.	13.4	2.0	12.0
SUN TOPS (Dole) any flavor	1 bar	Tr.		
SURIMI, *Crab Delights* (Louis Kemp) chunks, flakes or legs	2 oz.	Tr.		
SWAMP CABBAGE (USDA) boiled, trimmed, drained	4 oz.	.2		
SWEETBREADS (USDA):				
Beef, braised	4 oz.	26.3		

FOOD DESCRIPTION	MEASURE OR QUANTITY	Total	Saturated	Unsaturated
		FATS IN GRAMS		
Calf, braised	4 oz.	3.6		
Hog (See **PANCREAS**)				
Lamb, braised	4 oz.	6.9		
SWEET POTATO:				
Cooked (USDA) baked, peeled after baking	3.9-oz. potato (5″ × 2″)	.6		
Candied, home recipe (USDA)	6.2-oz. potato (3½″ × 2¼″)	0.0		
Canned (Joan of Arc) any style	½ cup	0.0		
Canned, dietetic pack (USDA) no added sugar or salt	4 oz.	.1		
Frozen (Mrs. Paul's) candied	⅓ of 12-oz. pkg.	Tr.		
SWEET POTATO PIE (USDA) home recipe, made with lard or vegetable shortening	⅙ of 9″ pie (5.4 oz.)	17.2	5.0	13.0
SWEET & SOUR CHICKEN (La Choy):				
*Canned, bi-pack	¾ cup	2.0		
Frozen	12-oz. entree	1.0		
SWEET & SOUR ORIENTAL, canned (La Choy):				
Chicken	¾ cup	2.0		
Pork	¾ cup	4.0		
SWORDFISH (USDA):				
Raw, meat only	1 lb.	18.1		
Broiled, with butter or margarine	3″ × 3″ × ½″ steak (4.4 oz.)	7.5		
SYRUP:				
Regular:				
Blackberry (Smucker's)	1 T.	0.0		
Blueberry (Smucker's)	1 T.	0.0		
Boysenberry (Smucker's)	1 T.	0.0		
Cane (USDA)	1 T.	0.0		
Chocolate:				
(USDA):				
Fudge type	1 T. (.7 oz.)	2.6	1.3	1.3
Thin type	1 T. (.7 oz.)	.4	.2	.2
(Hershey's)	1 T. (.5 oz.)	.5		
(Nestlé) *Quik*	1 oz.	0.0		
Corn, *Karo,* dark or light	1 T.	0.0		
Maple, *Karo,* imitation	1 T.	0.0		
Pancake or waffle:				
Log Cabin, any type	1 T.	0.0		
(Mrs. Butterworth's)	1 T.	.2		
Strawberry (Smucker's)	1 T.	0.0		
Dietetic:				
Chocolate (Estee)	1 T.	Tr.		
Pancake or waffle:				
(Mrs. Butterworth's)	1 T.	0.0		
(Weight Watchers)	1 T.	0.0		
TACO FILLING, canned (Old El Paso)	1 T.	1.0		
TACO SEASONING MIX (Lawry's)	1¼-oz. pkg.	1.1		
TACO SHELL:				
(Gebhardt)	.4-oz. shell	2.0		
(Old El Paso):				
Regular	1 shell	3.0		
Super	1 shell	6.0		
(Rosarita)	.4-oz. shell	2.0		
TACO BELL:				
Burrito:				
Bean, green or red sauce	6¾-oz. serving	10.2		
Beef, green or red sauce	6¾-oz. serving	17.3		
Supreme:				
Regular, green or red sauce	8½-oz. serving	17.5		
Double beef, green or red sauce	9-oz. serving	21.8		

FOOD DESCRIPTION	MEASURE OR QUANTITY	FATS IN GRAMS		
		Total	Saturated	Unsaturated
Cinnamon Crispas	1.7-oz. serving	15.3		
Enchirito, green or red sauce	7½-oz. serving	19.7		
Fajita:				
Chicken	4¾-oz. serving	10.2		
Steak	4¾-oz. serving	10.9		
Guacamole	¾-oz. serving	2.3		
Meximelt	3¾-oz. serving	15.4		
Nachos:				
Regular	3¾-oz. serving	18.5		
Bellgrande	10.1-oz. serving	35.3		
Pepper, jalapeño	3½-oz. serving	.2		
Pico De Gallo	1-oz. serving	.2		
Pintos & cheese, green or red sauce	4½-oz. serving	8.7		
Pizza, Mexican	7.9-oz. serving	36.8		
Ranch dressing	2.6-oz. serving	24.8		
Salsa	.3-oz. serving	.1		
Sour cream	¾-oz. serving	4.4		
Taco:				
Regular	2¾-oz. serving	10.8		
Bellgrande	5¾-oz. serving	23.1		
Light	6-oz. serving	28.8		
Soft:				
Regular	3¼-oz. serving	11.8		
Supreme	4.4-oz. serving	16.3		
Super combo	5-oz. serving	15.9		
Taco salad:				
Without shell	18.7-oz. serving	31.3		
With salsa:				
Regular	21-oz. serving	61.3		
Without shell	18.7-oz. serving	31.4		
Taco sauce, regular or hot	.4-oz. packet	Tr.		
Tostada, green or red sauce	5½-oz. serving	11.1		
TAMALE:				
Canned:				
(Old El Paso) with chili gravy	1 tamale	6.0		
(Pride of Mexico) beef	1 tamale (2 oz.)	8.5		
Frozen (Patio) dinner	13-oz. dinner	21.0		
TAMARIND, fresh (USDA) flesh only	4 oz.	.7		
TANG, instant breakfast drink, any flavor	6 fl. oz.	Tr.		
TANGELO, fresh (USDA) juice	½ cup (4.4 oz.)	.1		
TANGERINE OR MANDARIN ORANGE, fresh (USDA):				
Whole	5.1-oz. tangerine (2⅜" dia.)	.2		
Sections, without membranes	1 cup (6.8 oz.)	.4		
TANGERINE JUICE (USDA):				
Fresh	½ cup (4.4 oz.)	.2		
Canned, sweetened or unsweetened	½ cup (4.4 oz.)	.2		
*Frozen, prepared with 3 parts water by volume	½ cup (4.4 oz.)	.2		
TAPIOCA, dry, quick-cooking, granulated:				
(USDA)	1 cup (5.4 oz.)	.3		
(USDA)	1 T. (10 grams)	Tr.		
(Minute Tapioca)	1 T.	Tr.		
TAQUITO, frozen (Van de Kamp's) beef, shredded	8-oz. serving	25.0		
TARO (USDA):				
Tubers, skin removed	4 oz.	.2		
Leaves & stems	1 lb.	3.6		
TAUTOG OR BLACKFISH, raw (USDA) meat only	4 oz.	1.2		
TEA:				
Bag:				
*(Celestial Seasonings) any type	1 cup	Tr.		

FOOD DESCRIPTION	MEASURE OR QUANTITY	FATS IN GRAMS		
		Total	Saturated	Unsaturated
*(Lipton) regular, herbal or decaf	1 cup	0.0		
Instant:				
*(Lipton)	1 cup	0.0		
(Tender Leaf)	1 rounded tsp.	Tr.		
TEAM, cereal	1 cup (1 oz.)	1.0		
TEA, ICED, MIX:				
*All flavors (Salada)	1 cup	Tr.		
Lemon-flavored (Lipton) low-calorie	1 cup	Tr.		
TEENAGE MUTANT NINJA TURTLES, cereal (Ralston Purina)	1 cup (1 oz.)	0.0		
TEQUILA (See **DISTILLED LIQUOR**)				
TERIYAKI:				
*Canned (La Choy) chicken, bi-pack	¾ cup	2.0		
Frozen:				
(Armour) *Dinner Classics,* chicken	10½-oz. meal	15.0		
(Chun King)	13-oz. meal	2.0		
TERIYAKI BASTE & GLAZE OR SAUCE:				
(Kikkoman)	1 T.	Tr.		
(La Choy)	1 oz.	0.0		
TERRAPIN, DIAMOND BACK, raw (USDA) meat only	4 oz.	4.0		
TEXTURED VEGETABLE PROTEIN , *Morningstar Farms:*				
Breakfast links	1 link (.8 oz.)	5.7		
Breakfast patties	1 pattie (1.3 oz.)	7.2		
Breakfast slices	1 slice (1 oz.)	3.1	1.0	2.0
THURINGER, sausage:				
(USDA)	1 oz.	6.9		
(Eckrich), sliced or *Smoky Tang*	1 oz.	7.0		
(Hormel):				
Packaged, sliced	1 slice	5.5		
Whole:				
Regular or beefy	1 oz.	9.0		
Old Smokehouse	1 oz.	8.0		
(Oscar Mayer):				
Beef	.8-oz. slice	6.1	2.7	3.4
Meat	1-oz. slice	6.2	2.7	3.3
TILEFISH (USDA) baked, meat only	4 oz.	4.2		
TOPPING (See also **CHOCOLATE SYRUP**) sweetened:				
Butterscotch (Smucker's):				
Regular	1 T.	.5		
Special recipe	1 T.	1.5		
Caramel (Smucker's):				
Regular	1 T.	.5		
Hot	1 T.	2.0		
Chocolate:				
(Hershey's) fudge	1 T.	Tr.		
(Smucker's):				
Regular	1 T.	.5		
Fudge, hot	1 T.	2.0		
Nut (Planters)	1 T.	8.0		
Pecans, in syrup (Smucker's)	1 T.	.5		
Pineapple (Smucker's)	1 T.	0.0		
Peanut butter caramel (Smucker's)	1 T.	1.0		
Strawberry (Smucker's)	1 T.	0.0		
Walnuts in syrup (Smucker's)	1 T.	.5		
TOPPING, WHIPPED:				
(USDA):				
Pressurized	1 cup (2.5 oz.)	17.0	15.0	2.0
Pressurized	1 T. (4 grams)	1.0	Tr.	Tr.

FOOD DESCRIPTION	MEASURE OR QUANTITY	FATS IN GRAMS		
		Total	Saturated	Unsaturated
(Birds Eye) CoolWhip	1 T. (4 grams)	1.2		
La Creme (Pet)	1 T.	1.0		
TOPPING, WHIPPED, MIX:				
*(Dream Whip)	1 T. (.2 oz.)	.8		
*(Lucky Whip)	1 T. (4 grams)	6.0	Tr.	Tr.
TORTELLINI, frozen:				
(Buitoni):				
Cheese-filled, entree:				
Regular	2.6-oz. serving	6.3		
Tri-color	2.6-oz. serving	6.0		
Meat, plain	2.4-oz. serving	5.2	2.1	2.3
(Green Giant):				
Cheese marinara, one serving	5½-oz. pkg.	9.0		
Provencale, microwave	9½-oz. pkg.	5.0	1.0	1.0
(Stouffer's):				
Cheese:				
Alfredo sauce	8⅞-oz. serving	40.0		
Vinaigrette dressing	6⅞-oz. serving	27.0		
Veal, in alfredo sauce	8⅝-oz. serving	30.0		
TORTILLA (USDA)	7-oz. tortilla (5″)	.6		
TOSTADA, frozen (Van de Kamp's) beef	8½-oz. pkg.	30.0		
TOSTADA SHELL:				
(Old El Paso)	.4-oz. shell	3.2		
(Ortega)	.4-oz. shell	2.0		
TOTAL, cereal (General Mills) regular or corn	1 cup (1 oz.)	1.0		
TOWEL GOURD, raw (USDA) pared	4 oz.	.2		
TRIPE, beef (USDA):				
Commercial	4 oz.	2.3		
Pickled	4 oz.	1.5		
TROUT:				
Brook fresh (USDA) meat only	4 oz.	2.4		
Lake (See **LAKE TROUT**)				
Rainbow (USDA):				
Fresh, meat & skin	4 oz.	12.9	3.0	10.0
Canned	4 oz.	15.2	5.0	11.0
TUNA:				
Raw, meat only (USDA):				
Bluefin	4 oz.	4.6	1.0	4.0
Yellowfin, regular or brined	4 oz.	3.4	1.0	2.0
Canned in oil:				
Solids & liq.:				
(USDA)	6½-oz. can	37.7	9.0	29.0
(Breast O'Chicken)	6½-oz. can	36.8		
(Chicken of the Sea)	6-oz. can	25.6	3.0	22.0
Drained solids:				
(USDA)	6½-oz. can	27.7		
(Del Monte) albacore	1 cup (5.6 oz.)	13.1		
Canned in water:				
(USDA) solids & liq.	6½-oz. can	1.5		
(Breast O'Chicken)	6½-oz. can	1.8		
Canned, dietetic, drained, chunk, white (Chicken of the Sea)	6½-oz. can	2.6		
*TUNA HELPER** (General Mills):				
Au gratin or buttery rice	⅕ of pkg.	11.0		
Cheesy noodles	⅕ of pkg.	9.0		
Creamy noodles	⅕ of pkg.	14.0		
Tuna pot pie or tuna salad	⅕ of pkg.	27.0		
TUNA SALAD, home recipe (USDA)	4 oz.	11.9	3.0	9.0
TURBOT, GREENLAND, raw (USDA) meat only	4 oz.	9.5	2.0	8.0
TURKEY:				
Raw (USDA):				
Ready-to-cook	1 lb. (weighed with bones)	48.7	14.0	35.0

FOOD DESCRIPTION	MEASURE OR QUANTITY	FATS IN GRAMS		
		Total	Saturated	Unsaturated
Dark meat	4 oz.	4.9		
Light meat	4 oz.	1.4		
Skin only	4 oz.	44.5		
Roasted (USDA):				
Flesh, skin & giblets	From 13½-lb. raw, ready-to-cook turkey	603.5		
Flesh & skin	From 13½-lb. raw, ready-to-cook turkey	338.9	106.0	233.0
Meat only:				
Chopped	1 cup (5 oz.)	8.6	3.0	6.0
Dark	4 oz.	9.4	2.0	7.0
Dark	1 slice (2½" × 1⅝" × ¼", .7 oz.)	1.8	Tr.	1.0
Diced	1 cup (4.8 oz.)	8.2	3.0	6.0
Light	4 oz.	4.4	1.0	3.0
Light	1 slice (4" × 2" × ¼", 3 oz.)	1.7	Tr.	1.0
Skin only	1 oz.	11.9	3.0	9.0
Giblets, simmered (USDA)	2 oz.	8.7		
Canned, boned:				
(USDA)	4 oz.	14.2	5.0	10.0
(Swanson) with broth	5-oz. can	14.0		
Packaged:				
(Carl Buddig) smoked, sliced:				
Regular	1 oz.	3.0	1.0	2.0
Ham	1 oz.	.7	.7	
(Hormel) breast, regular or smoked	1 slice	1.0		
(Ohse):				
Oven cooked	1 oz.	1.0		
Turkey bologna	1 oz.	6.0		
Turkey salami	1 oz.	3.0		
(Oscar Mayer) breast, sliced:				
Oven roasted	.7-oz. slice	.5	.1	.3
Smoked	.7-oz. slice	.2	.1	.2
TURKEY DINNER OR ENTREE, (frozen):				
(Banquet)	10½-oz. dinner	20.0		
(Healthy Choice)	10½-oz. meal	5.0	2.0	1.0
(Stouffer's):				
Regular, casserole, with gravy & dressing	9¾-oz. meal	17.0		
Lean Cuisine:				
Breast, sliced, in mushroom sauce	8-oz. meal	7.0		
Dijon	9½-oz. meal	10.0		
Right Course, sliced, in mild curry sauce	8¾-oz. meal	8.0		
(Weight Watchers) stuffed breast	8½-oz. meal	10.0	4.0	6.0
TURKEY GIZZARD (USDA) simmered	4 oz.	9.8		
TURKEY PIE:				
Home recipe (USDA) baked	⅓ of 9" pie (8.2 oz.)	31.3	9.0	2.0
Frozen:				
(Empire Kosher)	8-oz. pie	24.0		
(Morton)	7-oz. pie	28.0		
(Stouffer's)	10-oz. pie	36.0		
TURKEY, POTTED (USDA)	1 oz.	5.4		
TURKEY SALAD, canned (Carnation) *Spreadables*	¼ of 7½-oz. can	7.5		
TURNIP (USDA):				
Fresh:				
Without tops	1 lb. (weighed with skins)	.8		
Pared, diced	½ cup (2.4 oz.)	.1		
Boiled, with or without salt, drained, diced or mashed	½ cup	.2		
TURNIP GREENS, leaves & stems:				
Boiled, drained (USDA)	½ cup (2.5 oz.)	.1		

FOOD DESCRIPTION	MEASURE OR QUANTITY	FATS IN GRAMS		
		Total	Saturated	Unsaturated
Canned, solids & liq.:				
(USDA)	½ cup (4.1 oz.)	.4		
(Stokely-Van Camp's)	½ cup (3.9 oz.)	.4		
Frozen (Birds Eye) chopped	½ cup (3.3 oz.)	.3		
TURNOVER:				
Frozen (Pepperidge Farm):				
Apple	3.1-oz. piece	17.0		
Blueberry or cherry	3.1-oz. piece	19.0		
Refrigerated (Pillsbury) apple or cherry	1 piece	8.0		
TURTLE, GREEN (USDA):				
Raw, meat only	4 oz.	.6		
Canned	4 oz.	.8		
ULTRA DIET QUICK (TKI Foods):				
Bar, chocolate or peanut butter	1.2-oz. bar	4.0		
*Mix, any flavor, made with water	8 fl. oz.	1.0		
VEAL, medium fat (USDA):				
Chuck, raw	1 lb. (weighed with bone)	36.0	17.0	19.0
Chuck, braised, lean & fat	4 oz.	14.5	7.0	8.0
Flank, raw	1 lb. (weighed with bone)	121.0	60.0	61.0
Flank, stewed, lean & fat	4 oz.	36.6	18.0	18.0
Foreshank, raw	1 lb. (weighed with bone)	19.0	10.0	9.0
Foreshank, stewed, lean & fat	4 oz.	11.8	6.0	6.0
Loin, raw	1 lb. (weighed with bone)	41.0	20.0	21.0
Loin, broiled, medium-done, chop, lean & fat	4 oz.	15.2	8.0	7.0
Plate, raw	1 lb. (weighed with bone)	61.0	30.0	31.0
Rib, raw, lean & fat	1 lb. (weighed with bone)	49.0	23.0	26.0
Rib, roasted, medium-done, lean & fat	4 oz.	19.2	9.0	10.0
Round & rump, raw	1 lb. (weighed with bone)	31.0	16.0	15.0
Round & rump, broiled, steak or cutlet, lean & fat	4 oz. (weighed without bone)	12.6	7.0	6.0
VEAL DINNER OR ENTREE, frozen:				
(Armour) *Dinner Classics,* parmigiana	11¼-oz. meal	22.0		
(Banquet) parmigiana:				
Cookin' bag, breaded	4-oz. pkg.	11.0		
Family Entree, patties	¼ of 32-oz. pkg.	18.0		
(Weight Watchers) parmigiana	8.4-oz. meal	10.0	3.0	7.0
VEGETABLE BOUILLON CUBE:				
(Herb-Ox)	1 cube (4 grams)	.1		
(Wyler's)	1 tsp.	Tr.		
VEGETABLE JUICE COCKTAIL, canned:				
(USDA)	4 oz. (by wt.)	.1		
V8 (Campbell's)	6 fl. oz.	0.0		
VEGETABLES, MIXED:				
Canned, solids & liq.:				
Regular pack:				
(Del Monte)	½ cup	Tr.		
(La Choy)	½ cup	Tr.		
Dietetic (Larsen) *Fresh-Lite*	½ cup	0.0		
Frozen:				
(Birds Eye):				
Regular:				
Broccoli, cauliflower & carrots in butter sauce	3.3 oz.	2.4		
Mixed	3.3 oz.	.4		
With onion sauce	⅓ of 8-oz. pkg.	5.3		

FOOD DESCRIPTION	MEASURE OR QUANTITY	FATS IN GRAMS		
		Total	Saturated	Unsaturated
Farm Fresh:				
Broccoli, corn & red pepper	1/5 of 16-oz. pkg.	Tr.		
Pea, carrot & pearl onion	1/5 of 16-oz. pkg.	Tr.		
(Green Giant):				
Broccoli, cauliflower & carrots:				
In butter sauce	1/3 of 9-oz. pkg.	1.0	Tr.	0.0
In cheese sauce	1/3 of 10-oz. pkg.	1.6	Tr.	Tr.
One serving:				
Plain	4-oz. pkg.	0.0		
Cheese sauce	5-oz. pkg.	3.0	Tr.	Tr.
Mixed, in butter sauce	1/2 cup	2.0	Tr.	0.0
Pea, sweet, carrot & pearl onion	1/2 cup	0.0		
(Le Sueur) pea, onion & carrot in butter sauce	1/2 cup	3.0		
(Larsen) regular, California, Italian or oriental blend	3.3 oz.	0.0		
(Ore-Ida):				
Medley, breaded	3 oz.	9.0	2.0	7.0
Stew	3 oz.	Tr.	Tr.	Tr.
"VEGETARIAN FOODS":				
Canned or dry:				
Chicken, fried (Loma Linda) with gravy	1 1/2-oz. piece	5.0		
Chili (Worthington)	1/2 cup	7.2		
Dinner cut (Loma Linda)	2.1-oz. piece	Tr.		
Franks (Loma Linda) big	1.8-oz. piece	5.0		
Frichick (Worthington)	1.6-oz. piece	4.5		
Gran Burger (Worthington)	1 oz.	.4		
Numete (Worthington)	1/2" slice	9.3		
Proteena (Loma Linda)	1/2" slice	6.0		
Redi-burger (Loma Linda)	1/2" slice	6.0		
Stew Pac (Loma Linda)	2 oz.	2.0		
Vege-Burger (Loma Linda)	1/2 cup	2.0		
Veg-scallops (Loma Linda)	1 piece	.2		
Frozen:				
Bologna (Loma Linda)	1-oz. slice	4.5		
Chicken, fried (Loma Linda)	2-oz. piece	14.0		
Chicken-like slices (Worthington)	1-oz. slice	2.8		
Chik-Nuggets (Loma Linda)	.6-oz. piece	2.2		
Corn dogs (Loma Linda)	2 1/2-oz. piece	19.0		
Meatballs (Loma Linda)	1 piece	1.0		
Meatless salami (Worthington)	3/4-oz. slice	2.2		
Olive loaf (Loma Linda)	1 slice	2.8		
Stripples (Worthington)	.3-oz. slice	1.3		
VENISON, raw, lean, meat only (USDA)	4 oz.	4.5	3.0	1.0
VERMOUTH, dry or sweet	Any quantity	0.0		
VINEGAR:				
Cider (USDA)	Any quantity	0.0		
Red or white wine (Regina)	1 T.	Tr.		
VINESPINACH OR BASELLA, raw (USDA)	4 oz.	.3		
VODKA, unflavored (See **DISTILLED LIQUOR**)				
WAFFLE:				
Home recipe (USDA)	2.6-oz. waffle (7" dia.)	7.4	2.0	5.0
Frozen:				
(Aunt Jemima) original	1 section (3/4 oz.)	2.4		
(Eggo):				
Regular	1.4-oz. waffle	5.0	1.0	4.0
Common Sense, oat bran:				
Plain	1.4-oz. waffle	4.0	1.0	3.0
With fruit & nuts	1.4-oz. waffle	5.0	1.0	4.0

FOOD DESCRIPTION	MEASURE OR QUANTITY	FATS IN GRAMS		
		Total	Saturated	Unsaturated
Nutri-Grain, plain or raisin & bran	1.4-oz. waffle	5.0	1.0	4.0
WAFFLE MIX (USDA) (See also **PANCAKE & WAFFLE MIX**):				
Dry, complete mix	1 oz.	5.4	1.0	4.0
*Prepared with water	2.6-oz. waffle (1/2" × 41/2" × 51/2", 7" dia.)	10.5	2.0	8.0
Dry, incomplete mix	1 oz.	.5		
*Prepared with egg & milk	2.6-oz. waffle (7" dia.)	8.0	3.0	5.0
WAFFLE SYRUP (See **SYRUP**)				
WALNUT (USDA):				
Black:				
Shelled, whole	4 oz.	67.2	5.0	63.0
Chopped	1/2 cup (2.1 oz.)	35.6	2.0	33.0
English or Persian:				
Shelled, whole	4 oz.	72.6	4.5	68.0
Chopped	1/2 cup (2.1 oz.)	38.4	2.0	36.0
WATER CHESTNUT, CHINESE, raw (USDA):				
Whole	1 lb. (weighed unpeeled)	.7		
Peeled	4 oz.	.2		
WATERCRESS, raw (USDA) trimmed	1/2 cup (.6 oz.)	Tr.		
WATERMELON, fresh (USDA):				
Whole	1 lb. (weighed with rind)	.4		
Diced	1 cup (5.6 oz.)	.3		
WAX GOURD, raw (USDA) flesh only	4 oz.	.2		
WEAKFISH (USDA) broiled, meat only	4 oz.	12.9		
WELSH RAREBIT:				
Home recipe (USDA)	1 cup (8.2 oz.)	31.6	16.0	15.0
Canned (Snow's)	4 oz.	11.4		
Frozen (Stouffer's)	5 oz.	29.0		
WENDY'S:				
Bacon, breakfast	1 strip	5.0		
Bacon cheeseburger	5.2-oz. serving	28.0		
Breakfast sandwich	4.5-oz. sandwich	19.0		
Buns:				
Wheat, multi-grain	1.7-oz. piece	3.0		
White	1.8-oz. piece	3.0		
Chicken sandwich on wheat bun	41/2-oz. sandwich	10.0		
Chili	8-oz. serving	8.0		
Condiments:				
Bacon	1/2 strip	2.7		
Cheese, American	.6-oz. slice	6.0		
Ketchup	1 tsp.	Tr.		
Lettuce	1 piece	Tr.		
Mayonnaise	1 T.	11.0		
Mustard	1 tsp.	Tr.		
Onions	.3-oz. piece	Tr.		
Pickles, dill	4 slices	Tr.		
Relish	.3-oz. serving	Tr.		
Tomatoes	1 slice	Tr.		
Danish	3-oz. piece	18.0		
Drinks:				
Cola:				
Regular	12 fl. oz.	Tr.		
Dietetic	12 fl. oz.	Tr.		
Fruit flavored	12 fl. oz.	Tr.		
Hot chocolate	6 fl. oz.	3.0		
Milk:				
Regular	8 fl. oz.	8.0		
Chocolate	8 fl. oz.	8.0		
Orange juice	6 fl. oz.	Tr.		
Tea:				
Hot	6 fl. oz.	Tr.		
Iced	12 fl. oz.	Tr.		
Eggs, scrambled	3.2-oz. serving	12.0		

FOOD DESCRIPTION	MEASURE OR QUANTITY	FATS IN GRAMS		
		Total	Saturated	Unsaturated
Hamburgers:				
Double, on white bun	7-oz. serving	34.0		
Kids meal	2.6-oz. serving	8.0		
Single:				
On wheat bun	4.2-oz. serving	17.0		
On white bun	4.2-oz. serving	18.0		
Omelets:				
Ham & cheese	1 omelet	17.0		
Ham, cheese, onion & green pepper	1 omelet	19.0		
Mushroom, onion & green pepper	1 omelet	15.0		
Potatoes:				
Baked, hot stuffed:				
Plain	8.8-oz. potato	2.0		
Broccoli & cheese	12.9-oz. potato	25.0		
Chili & cheese	14.1-oz. potato	20.0		
Sour cream & chives	10.9-oz. potato	24.0		
French fries	3½-oz. serving	14.0		
Home fries	2.6-oz. serving	22.0		
Salad bar:				
Alfalfa sprouts	2 oz.	Tr.		
Bacon bits	⅛ oz.	Tr.		
Blueberries	1 T.	Tr.		
Breadsticks	1 piece	1.0		
Broccoli	½ cup (1.6 oz.)	Tr.		
Cantaloupe	2 pieces (2 oz.)	0.0		
Carrots	¼ cup (1 oz.)	Tr.		
Cauliflower	½ cup (1.8 oz.)	Tr.		
Cheese:				
American	1 oz.	5.0		
Cottage	½ cup	6.0		
Mozzarella	1 oz.	7.0		
Swiss	1 oz.	6.0		
Chow mein noodles	¼ cup	3.0		
Cole slaw	½ cup	8.0		
Crackers, saltine	1 piece	.5		
Croutons	1 piece	.1		
Cucumber	¼ cup	Tr.		
Mushrooms	¼ cup (.6 oz.)	Tr.		
Onions, red	1 T.	Tr.		
Pasta salad	½ cup (3.5 oz.)	6.0		
Peas, green	½ cup (2.8 oz.)	Tr.		
Pineapple chunks in juice	½ cup	Tr.		
Watermelon	1 piece (1 oz.)	Tr.		
Salad dressing:				
Regular:				
Blue cheese	1 T.	7.0		
French, red	1 T.	5.0		
Italian, golden	1 T.	4.0		
Ranch	1 T.	9.0		
Dietetic:				
Bacon & tomato	1 T.	4.0		
Italian	1 T.	2.0		
Thousand island	1 T.	4.0		
Wine vinegar	1 T.	Tr.		
Sausage patty	1.6-oz. patty	18.0		
Toast:				
Regular, with margarine	1.2-oz. slice	4.5		
French	2.4-oz. slice	9.5		
WESTERN DINNER, frozen:				
(Banquet)	11-oz. dinner	41.0		
(Morton)	10-oz. dinner	14.0		
WEST INDIAN CHERRY (See ACEROLA)				
WHALE MEAT raw (USDA)	4 oz.	8.5	1.0	7.0
WHEAT FLAKES, cereal (USDA) crushed	1 cup (2.5 oz.)	1.1		
WHEAT GERM, crude, commercial, milled (USDA)	1 oz.	3.1	Tr.	3.0

FOOD DESCRIPTION	MEASURE OR QUANTITY	FATS IN GRAMS		
		Total	Saturated	Unsaturated
WHEAT GERM CEREAL:				
(USDA)	¼ cup (1 oz.)	3.2	Tr.	3.0
(Kretschmer):				
Regular	¼ cup (1 oz.)	3.1		
With sugar & honey	¼ cup (1 oz.)	2.3		
WHEAT HEARTS, cereal				
(General Mills) dry, hot	1 oz. (3⅓ T.)	1.0		
WHEATIES, cereal (General				
Mills)	1 cup (1 oz.)	1.0		
WHEAT, PUFFED, cereal:				
(Post) super golden crisp	⅞ cup	Tr.		
(Sunland)	½ oz.	3.0		
WHEAT, ROLLED (USDA):				
Uncooked	1 cup (3.1 oz.)	1.7		
Cooked, salt added	1 cup (7.7 oz.)	.9		
WHEAT, SHREDDED, cereal				
(See **SHREDDED WHEAT**)				
WHEY, fluid (USDA)	1 cup (8.6 oz.)	.7		
WHISKY OR WHISKEY (See				
DISTILLED LIQUOR)				
WHITE CASTLE:				
Bun	.9-oz. bun	.9		
Cheese	.3-oz. piece	1.6		
Cheeseburger	2.3-oz. serving	11.2		
Chicken sandwich	2¼-oz. serving	7.4		
Fish sandwich, without tartar				
sauce	2.1-oz. sandwich	5.0		
French fries	1 order	14.7		
Hamburger	2.1-oz. burger	7.9		
Onion chips	3.3-oz. order	16.5		
Onion rings	1 order	13.4		
Sausage & egg sandwich	3.4-oz. sandwich	22.0		
Sausage sandwich	1.7-oz. sandwich	12.3		
WHITEFISH, LAKE (USDA):				
Raw, meat only	4 oz.	9.3		
Baked, stuffed, home recipe	4 oz.	15.9		
Smoked	4 oz.	8.3		
WHITEFISH & PIKE (See				
GEFILTE FISH)				
WILD RICE, raw (USDA)	½ cup (2.9 oz.)	.6		
WINE	Any quantity	0.0		
WINE COOLER (Bartles &				
Jaymes) any flavor	6 fl. oz.	0.0		
WORCESTERSHIRE SAUCE				
(See **SAUCE,** Worcestershire)				
WRECKFISH, raw, meat only				
(USDA)	4 oz.	4.4		
YAM (USDA):				
Raw, flesh only	4 oz.	.2		
Canned & frozen (See **SWEET**				
POTATO)				
YAM BEAN (USDA) raw, pared				
tuber	4 oz.	.2		
YEAST:				
Baker's:				
Compressed (USDA)	1 oz.	.1		
Dry (Fleischmann's)	¼-oz. (pkg. or jar)	.1		
Brewer's dry, debittered				
(USDA)	1 oz.	.3		
YELLOWTAIL, raw, meat only				
(USDA)	4 oz.	6.1		
YOGURT:				
Made from whole milk				
(USDA)	½ cup (4.3 oz.)	4.1	2.0	2.0
Made from partially skimmed				
milk, plain or vanilla				
(USDA)	8-oz. container	3.9	2.0	2.0
Made from partially skimmed				
milk, fruit-flavored (USDA)	8-oz. container	2.7		

FOOD DESCRIPTION	MEASURE OR QUANTITY	FATS IN GRAMS		
		Total	Saturated	Unsaturated
Regular:				
Plain:				
(Dannon):				
Low-fat	8-oz. container	4.0		
Nonfat	8-oz. container	0.0		
(Friendship)	8-oz. container	3.0		
(Johanna) sundae style	8-oz. container	4.0		
Lite-Line (Borden)	8-oz. container	2.0		
Yoplait (General Mills):				
Regular	6-oz. container	3.0		
Nonfat	8-oz. serving	0.0		
Apple (Dannon) dutch, fruit-on-the-bottom	8-oz. container	3.0		
Banana:				
(Dannon) fruit-on-the-bottom	8-oz. container	3.0		
Yoplait (General Mills)	6-oz. container	3.0		
Banana-strawberry (Colombo)	8-oz. container	6.0		
Berry, Yoplait (General Mills) mixed:				
Regular or Breakfast Yogurt	6-oz. container	3.0		
Custard Style	6-oz. container	4.0		
Blueberry:				
(Dannon):				
Fresh Flavors	8-oz. container	4.0		
Fruit-on-the-bottom:				
Small	4.4-oz. container	2.0		
Regular	8-oz. container	3.0		
Yoplait (General Mills):				
Regular	6-oz. container	3.0		
Light	6-oz. container	0.0		
Boysenberry (Dannon) fruit-on-the-bottom	8-oz. container	3.0		
Cherry:				
(Dannon) fruit-on-the-bottom	8-oz. container	3.0		
Yoplait (General Mills):				
Breakfast Yogurt, with almonds	6-oz. container	3.0	2.0	1.0
Light	6-oz. container	0.0		
Cherry-vanilla, Lite-Line (Borden)	8-oz. container	2.0		
Coffee:				
(Friendship)	8-oz. container	3.0		
(Johanna) sundae-style	8-oz. container	4.0		
Exotic fruit (Dannon) fruit-on-the-bottom	8-oz. container	3.0		
Lemon:				
(Dannon) Fresh Flavors	8-oz. container	3.0		
Yoplait (General Mills):				
Regular	6-oz. container	3.0		
Custard Style	6-oz. container	4.0		
Mixed berries (Dannon):				
Extra smooth	4.4-oz. serving	2.0		
Fruit-on-the-bottom	8-oz. container	3.0		
Orange, Yoplait (General Mills):				
Regular	6-oz. container	3.0		
Custard Style	6-oz. container	4.0		
Peach:				
(Dannon) fruit-on-the-bottom	8-oz. container	3.0		
(Whitney's)	6-oz. container	5.0		
Pina colada:				
(Dannon) fruit-on-the-bottom	8-oz. container	3.0		

FOOD DESCRIPTION	MEASURE OR QUANTITY	FATS IN GRAMS		
		Total	Saturated	Unsaturated
Yoplait (General Mills):				
Regular	6-oz. container	3.0		
Custard Style	5-oz. container	4.0		
Pineapple, *Yoplait* (General Mills)	8-oz. container	3.0		
Raspberry:				
(Dannon):				
Extra smooth	4.4-oz. container	2.0		
Fresh Flavors	8-oz. container	4.0		
(Whitney's)	6-oz. container	5.0		
Yoplait (General Mills):				
Regular	6-oz. container	3.0		
Light	6-oz. container	0.0		
Strawberry:				
(Dannon):				
Extra smooth	4.4-oz. container	2.0		
Fruit-on-the-bottom	4.4-oz. container	2.0		
Light	8-oz. container	0.0		
Lite-Line (Borden)	8-oz. container	2.0		
(Whitney's)	6-oz. container	5.0		
Yoplait (General Mills):				
Regular	6-oz. container	3.0		
Breakfast Yogurt, with almonds	6-oz. container	3.0	2.0	1.0
Custard Style	4-oz. container	3.0		
Light	6-oz. container	0.0		
Strawberry-banana:				
(Whitney's)	6-oz. container	5.0		
Yoplait (General Mills):				
Regular	6-oz. container	3.0		
Breakfast Yogurt	6-oz. container	3.0	1.0	2.0
Custard Style	6-oz. container	4.0		
Light	6-oz. container	0.0		
Strawberry-rhubarb, *Yoplait* (General Mills)	6-oz. container	3.0		
Tropical fruits:				
(Whitney's)	6-oz. container	6.0		
Yoplait (General Mills)				
Breakfast Yogurt	6-oz. container	4.0		
Vanilla:				
(Dannon) light, regular or cherry	8-oz. container	0.0		
(Friendship)	8-oz. container	3.0		
(Whitney's)	6-oz. container	6.0		
Yoplait (General Mills):				
Custard Style	6-oz. container	4.0		
Nonfat	8-oz. container	0.0		
Frozen, soft serve (Baskin-Robbins):				
Banana or cheesecake	1 fl. oz.	.4		
Chocolate	1 fl. oz.	.6		
Coconut	1 fl. oz.	1.0		
YOGURT BAR, frozen (Dole) any flavor	1 bar	Tr.		
ZINFANDEL WINE	Any quantity	0.0		
ZINGERS (Dolly Madison):				
Devil's food or raspberry	1¼-oz. piece	5.0		
White	1¼-oz. piece	4.0		
ZWIEBACK:				
(USDA)	1 oz.	2.5	.6	1.9
(Nabisco)	¼-oz. piece	.5	Tr.	Tr.

ABOUT THE AUTHOR

Barbara Kraus, noted cook and food authority, won instant acclaim with her best-seller *Calories and Carbohydrates,* and her pioneering work *The Dictionary of Sodium, Fats, and Cholesterol.* She is credited with helping arouse public consciousness of the importance of eating both well and wisely. Her master's degree in anthropology focused largely on the cultural aspects of food uses and cooking habits. Her many works include the popular cookbooks *The Cookbook of the United Nations* and *The Cookbook to Serve 2, 6, or 24.*

BIBLIOGRAPHY

Reusch, H. *Top of the World.* New York: Pocket Books, 1969.
USDA Handbook No. 8, *Composition of Foods.*

Nutrition titles from Perigree, by the foremost experts in the field!

These books are available at your local bookstore or wherever books are sold. Ordering is also easy and convenient. Just call 1-800-631-8571, or send your order to:

The Putnam Publishing Group
390 Murray Hill Parkway, Dept. B
East Rutherford, NJ 07073

		Price U.S.	Canada
____ The Barbara Kraus Calorie Counter	399-51222-5	$ 6.95	$ 9.25
____ The Barbara Kraus Cholesterol Counter	399-51134-2	6.95	9.25
____ The Barbara Kraus Fat Counter	399-51715-4	7.95	10.50
____ The Barbara Kraus International Cookbook	399-51655-7	14.95	19.50
____ The Barbara Kraus 30-Day Cholesterol Program	399-51508-9	6.95	9.25
____ Carlton Fredericks' New Low Blood Sugar and You	399-51087-7	7.95	10.50
____ Carlton Fredericks' Sodium Counter	399-51509-7	6.95	9.25
____ Dictionary of Sodium, Fats, and Cholesterol, 2nd ed.	399-51572-0	12.95	16.95
____ Dr. Bruce Lowell's Fat % Finder	399-51653-0	8.95	11.75
____ Lower Your Cholesterol in 30 Days	399-51555-0	4.95	6.50

Subtotal $_____

Postage & handling* $_____

Sales Tax (CA, NJ, NY, PA) $_____

Total Amount Due $_____

Payable in U.S. Funds (no cash orders accepted). $10.00 minimum for credit card orders.

*Postage & handling: $2.00 for 1 book, 50¢ for each additional book up to a maximum of $4.50.

Enclosed is my ☐ check ☐ money order
Please charge my ☐ Visa ☐ MasterCard ☐ American Express
Card # _____ Expiration date _____

Signature as on charge card _____

Name _____

Address _____

City _____ State _____ Zip _____

Please allow six weeks for delivery. Prices subject to change without notice.